THE EVALU FOR HEALTH PROFESSIO

For the growing number of health professionals who are engaged in processes of evaluation in a variety of contexts within the world of healthcare, *The Evaluation Handbook* is an easy-to-use resource. Encouraging an evidence-based approach to practice, it provides:

- guidelines on how to design and evaluate an intervention
- examples of good practice
- reliable and easy-to-use measures
- advice on how to work effectively.

The handbook is designed to prompt self-evaluation and group project evaluation. It illustrates how simple evaluation methods can help to break down the divisions between research and practice and how more practitioners can apply such methods to improve the quality of care as well as the treatments and services which they offer their patients and clients. The examples, drawn from clinical settings, community practice and work in the voluntary sector, illustrate the kind of evaluation that can be undertaken by a small-scale team or a single practitioner with limited resources.

The Evaluation Handbook will be a useful source of reference for those new to evaluation as well as more experienced managers and researchers.

Anne Lazenbatt is a Reader in Health Sciences and Associate Head of the School of Nursing and Midwifery at The Queen's University of Belfast.

THE EVALUATION HANDBOOK FOR HEALTH PROFESSSIONALS

Anne Lazenbatt

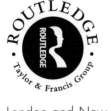

London and New York

First published 2002
by Routledge
11 New Fetter Lane, London EC4P 4EE

Simultaneously published in the USA and Canada
by Routledge
29 West 35th Street, New York, NY 10001

Routledge is an imprint of the Taylor & Francis Group

Designed and typeset in Sabon and Futura by
Keystroke, Jacaranda Lodge, Wolverhampton
Printed and bound in Great Britain by
TJ International Ltd, Padstow, Cornwall

British Library Cataloguing in Publication Data
A catalogue record for this book is available from the British Library

Library of Congress Cataloging in Publication Data
Lazenbatt, Anne, 1953–
The evaluation handbook for health professional / Anne Lazenbatt.
p. cm.
Includes bibliographical references and index.
1. Medical care—Evaluation—Handbooks, manuals, etc. I. Title.

RA399.A1 L39 2002
362.1'068'5—dc21   2001048590

ISBN 0–415–24857–4 (hbk)
ISBN 0–415–24858–2 (pbk)

CONTENTS

FIGURES AND TABLES

FIGURES

TABLES

CHAPTER 1

INTRODUCTION

INTRODUCTION

It is now widely recognized that an understanding of evaluation methodology is essential for all nursing and healthcare professionals. It is necessary for nurses, midwives and health visitors to be able to evaluate their own practice and the practice of others. Not all practitioners will want to become researchers; however, they should be able to appreciate the evaluation methods of others and understand how to incorporate evaluation findings into their own professional practice. All practitioners are being encouraged to stand back and reflect on the services they are providing. They must question the evidence base for these services and ask whether the delivery of these services is efficient and effective for the communities and individuals they serve. The criteria for evaluation of health, social, environmental and economic policies and programmes are changing. Many governments are now adopting an understanding of health that embraces issues of equity and inequality and the significance of social and environmental determinants. Without tools and methods to assess the health impact of policies and programmes we cannot assess which strategies work best to achieve beneficial outcomes.

This handbook is designed to meet the needs of the growing number of health professionals who are engaged in processes of evaluation in a variety of contexts within the world of healthcare and to assist in the development of an environment which fosters the monitoring and assessment of practice within the nursing and health professions to include:

- the development of a culture where practitioners question the appropriateness of their interventions and where evaluation of practice is considered a regular aspect of care delivery
- the provision of further training and education in the techniques involved in research and evaluation.

Since definition by example is often the most effective way of communicating information, the handbook is based around a number of illustrative case studies which will hopefully encourage a research evidence-based approach to evaluation by offering guidelines for those wishing to design and evaluate an intervention; offering standards of measurement of process, patient/client satisfaction and patient/client focused outcomes assessment; and illustrating multidisciplinary effectiveness and collaborative work with other agencies.

As the recent founding of the National Institute for Clinical Excellence (NICE) suggests, in the future such concepts as clinical governance and health impact assessment will become increasingly important in providing standards of quality assurance within the health professions. For instance, clinical governance will involve health professionals wanting to assure the quality and accountability of their healthcare delivery. This will require staff not only to work in partnerships, breaking down boundaries by providing integrated care within health and social care teams but also to participate fully in audit and evaluation programmes. It will strengthen the current systems of quality assurance, as it will be based upon the evaluation of clinical standards, better utilization of evidence-based practice and lessons learnt from poor performance.

To assist practitioners the handbook places emphasis on evaluation processes and measures which are easy to use and are seen as an integral part of quality improvement. Healthcare staff of the future must be able to shape their healthcare delivery systems and plan change through good models of evaluation, open communication, collaboration, health impact assessment and improved client and patient health and social care. Health impact assessment (HIA) has been defined as 'any combination of procedures or methods by which proposed policy or programmes may be judged as to the effects it may have on the health of the population' (Lock, 2000). With increasing commitment to community participation in decision-making and the growing consideration of the social and environmental determinants of health there is a growing controversy about what impact on health these new perspectives will have. In recognizing the complexity and potentially far-reaching effects of many policies and programmes, desirable assessments should therefore involve intersectoral partnerships and collaboration as well as lay experiences.

Chapter 2 concentrates on promotion of health and wellbeing within an inequalities framework. As it is now widely accepted that the determinants of health inequalities lie outside the health sector the greatest scope for improving the public's health requires the growth of new policies beyond this sector. Health impact assessment has emerged to identify those activities and policies likely to have major impacts on the health of a population. Building healthy public policy was a key component of the Ottawa Charter for health promotion (WHO, 1986) so we can see that the basic concepts of HIA are not new. The UK government has only recently explicitly acknowledged a need to assess how all public policy are impacting on health. The three public health consultative documents for Northern Ireland, Wales and Scotland and the English public health white paper have all referred to the requirement for health impact assessment of both national and local policies and projects (Secretary of State Northern Ireland, 1997; Secretary of State for Wales, 1998; Secretary of State for Scotland, 1999; Secretary of State for Health, 1999). Health impact assessment should therefore be thought of as a group of research and evaluation activities being developed to identify health impacts of projects and policies both prospectively and retrospectively. It is a structured way of bringing together evaluation, partnership working, public consultation and indicators such as medical, surgical and nursing outcomes, quality assurance and utilization indicators, as well as available evidence for more explicit decision-making. We now need to know which strategies work best to achieve beneficial outcomes for patients and communities. It is hoped that this handbook will play its own part in assisting practitioners, policy-makers and different population groups towards that goal. We return to the issues of clinical governance and health impact assessment in Chapter 3.

The handbook illustrates how evaluation is an extension of what we all do in everyday life: when we want to know answers we ask questions and we evaluate the information we are given before making use of it. Good evaluation has been defined as using 'the methodological imagination' (Nutbeam and Wise, 1996). This means that it is not enough just to collect data; we also need to think long and hard about the nature of the intervention, the methodologies that we use, and the part evaluation plays in shaping and interpreting it, what it means to consumers and participants and what is needed to improve it.

Chapters 10–13 of this handbook provide a collection of examples of evaluation techniques, all concerned in some way with nursing or the study of health and community care. Evidence-based practice is now seen as central to the development of nursing as a profession. Each evaluation covers the various stages of evaluation; namely, needs assessment, structure, process and outome. The examples are intended to illustrate the kinds of evaluation that can be undertaken by a small-scale evaluation team or by a single practitioner with limited resources to investigate various aspects of practice in the clinical field, within the community and in the voluntary sector. The four stages utilize a diversity of qualitative and quantitative methods and each reflects the experience of applied evaluation as it occurs in practice, as opposed to how it tends to look in textbooks. In Chapter 4 the handbook offers a collection of shorter case studies that illustrate examples of 'best' practice in the area of inequalities in health and social need.

WHAT IS THE HANDBOOK ABOUT?

Health practitioners need an easy-to-use handbook that provides information about reliable indicators and tools for evaluation, especially for the measurement of a holistic view of health. This handbook attempts to meet that need by offering a working resource for all those involved in health education and in the promotion of health and social wellbeing within the area of inequalities in health. Chapter 2 deals with aspects of how we can target and attempt to tackle inequalities in health and the issues surrounding equity in healthcare. However, it must be stressed that the handbook can be used by those new to evaluation and those wishing to apply it to areas beyond inequalities in health. It is designed as a tool that will prompt self-evaluation and group project evaluation. It uses a pluralistic and practical approach because the subject deals with the evaluation of health and social interventions of many different types. Both evaluators and users of evaluations need to know which type of evaluation could be used and the advantages and limitations of each. The evaluation of health and social need interventions raises questions about our own and others' values. It involves issues about how we might change clinical, community and managerial practice and about how governments and organizations make health policies that affect us all. Chapter 4 highlights eight case examples of 'quality' interventions from community and hospital-based perspectives. These illustrate how simple evaluation methods may help to break down the divisions between research and practice and how more practitioners are applying such methods to improve the quality of care as well as the treatments and services that they offer their patients and clients. Chapter 5 gives a broad introduction to evaluation while Chapter 6 sets out the planning process required before you embark on your evaluation.

Since interventions which tackle inequalities in health may vary enormously in size and complexity, the appropriate evaluation must be tailored to fit their needs. At one end of the scale are small evaluations involving a single practitioner working without the advantage of funding; at the other end evaluations may be undertaken by multi-disciplinary teams, lasting several years with a large budget and often with tight contractual obligations to their funding bodies. Although the problems of management are more complex in larger evaluations, the issues and principles remain the same irrespective of size. This handbook aligns itself with a more 'pluralistic' view of evaluation; however, it does not criticize alternative styles and the reader should be aware that each approach can inform the other and has its place. As stated, although different approaches are required for the many types of intervention that need to be evaluated there is plenty of room for all in this new and growing field.

WHO IS THE HANDBOOK FOR?

The handbook is designed to assist those who are planning an evaluation or those who are already working on an evaluation – this includes health alliances, multidisciplinary teams, and all those agencies collaborating and working together with the statutory, private, community and voluntary sectors. It is expected that it should prove useful to nurses and midwives, clinicians and general practitioners, PAMS, teachers, and other professionals working within health and social need. The handbook is also for managers, advisors and policy-makers who use or sponsor evaluations: they are defined as 'users' as are practitioners and, increasingly, patients, clients and lay health workers. The book is not intended to be prescriptive but to serve as an aid to evaluation. All health professionals, whatever their position in work, need to understand the fundamentals of evaluation. They will need even more in the future to be able to apply findings from evaluations, and to use evaluation methods to improve their own clinical, community or managerial practice and the surrounding organization of care.

AIMS

Chapters 7–9 of the handbook aim to offer a step-by-step pathway through the 'pluralistic' method necessary in order to assess processes and outcomes in such complex evaluations. It will demonstrate that such questions as 'How do we know that interventions work?' and 'How do they succeed, where do they fail and do they remain effective over time?' require a multi-method approach if they are to be given satisfactory answers. It will also give guidance about the meaning of success by setting out the main evidence from systematic reviews and from the demonstrated evidence of best practice in the area. Each chapter in the handbook provides details of further and recommended reading to allow readers to expand their knowledge and competence about the new terminology.

FURTHER READING

Lock, K. (2000) Health impact assessment. *British Medical Journal*, 320: 1395–1398.

Nutbeam, D. and Wise, M. (1996) Planning for health for all: international experience in setting health goals and targets. *Health Promotion International*, 11(3): 219–226.

Secretary of State for Northern Ireland (1997) *Well into 2000*. Belfast: Department of Health and Social Services.

Secretary of State for Scotland (1999) *Towards a Healthier Scotland*. Edinburgh: Stationery Office.

Secretary of State for Wales (1998) *Better health better Wales*. London: Stationery Office.

Secretary of State for Health (1999) *Saving Lives: Our Healthier Nation*. London: Stationery Office.

World Health Organisation (1986) *The Ottawa Charter: Principles for Health Promotion*. Copenhagen: WHO regional office for Europe.

PART ONE

CHAPTER 2

INEQUALITIES IN HEALTH

TARGETING HEALTH AND SOCIAL NEED

Health inequalities have been documented in Britain for over a hundred years indeed, and recent evidence suggests that they are actually widening (Whitehead *et al.*, 2000). In the last few decades, almost all developed countries have found that disadvantaged groups are more likely to die young and have more illness than more affluent groups (Benzeval, 1998). We know then that inequalities in health and social wellbeing exist and the current debate today is what can be done about these inequalities in both health and social need. The publication of the Black Report (Black *et al.*, 1980) and *The Health Divide* (Whitehead, 1987) represented new landmarks in our knowledge and understanding of inequalities in health. Twenty years ago the Secretary of State for Social Services of the last Labour Government appointed Sir Douglas Black to chair a working group on inequalities in health and suggest policy and research that should follow from this review. The report appeared in 1980 and received a cold reception from the new Conservative government. In 1985, the British Government signed the WHO's *Health for All Charter* but again did little until the 1990s when in 1992 the *Health of the Nation* White Paper was published (DoH, 1992). Disappointingly, this document had little focus, as it was lifestyle-orientated and failed to address health inequalities, only briefly discussing 'variations' in health. However, in 1995 the King's Fund developed an impressive agenda for action that covered a broad range of social policies designed to tackle health inequalities (Benzeval *et al.*, 1995).

The climate for the Black report's successor – the *Independent Inquiry into Inequalities in Health*, chaired by Sir Donald Acheson and published in 1998 – is hopefully different. This much-awaited report heralds evidence from an impressive list of institutional and individual contributors and synthesizes this into a comprehensive review of the current knowledge on the extent and trends of inequalities in health and the determinants of health in the UK today. It stresses the increasing inequalities in income that have left the United Kingdom leading the developed world in income inequality and child poverty. The first of its 39 recommendations calls for an assessment of all policies likely to have an impact on inequalities in health. Internationally, the World Health Organisation (WHO), the World Bank (1997) and the European Union (EU) are calling for health impact assessments of all programmes and policies. New health strategies have recently been launched in the UK around the twin goals of improving population health and narrowing 'the health gap in childhood and through-out life between socio-economic groups' (Secretary of State for Health, 2000). The new public health strategies have mostly been structured around health improvement targets: with targets being set to reduce mortality and morbidity rates from cancer, coronary heart disease, suicide and accidents. In February 2001, the Government carried through the commitment made in the *NHS Plan* to underwrite health inequality targets with national targets (DoH, 2001).

We know that there is a lot to be done. We need to promote community needs and health needs assessments, health profiling, health impact assessments and equity audits, and evaluate our interventions so that we can understand what it is that we are doing that is inequitable and how we can tackle it. We need to empower communities and individuals to define their own problems and together with them begin to develop strategies and solutions to these problems. Practitioners need to understand the social context of illness and ensure that healthcare becomes more culturally sensitive, services are targeted and reach out to those who need them. Community practitioners and health visitors have a vital role to play in the creation of organizations and systems that promote equity and health that is central to the NHS and to work with communities to identify their problems and address them.

The concepts of social class, poverty, socio-economic status and deprivation have all been used at various times to explain and theorize about inequalities in health. They are widespread phenomena resulting from a complex interplay of many different factors such as gender, age, race, community background, ill health and disability, lack of education, unemployment, poor housing and lack of social support. Health promoters sometimes feel powerless to effect change on such a fundamental level but the nursing community has shown how they are producing changes in practice which acknowledge social conditions and social wellbeing (Lazenbatt, 1997, 1999; Lazenbatt and Orr, 2001).

This handbook describes examples of nursing and midwifery interventions that reflect the difficulties many people face in securing the basic resources which provide the necessary foundation for reasonable health, i.e. shelter, warmth, food, social interaction and personal care. In describing their work, they reflect in detail the impact of poverty on people's health such as the lack of good quality housing, leisure facilities, access to health and social services and reduced opportunities for education and employment. The accounts illustrate the interactive nature of psychological and physical wellbeing, and contribute to our growing evidence base which suggests that lack of the material resources necessary to promote or maintain health negatively affects emotional as well as physical health (Blaxter, 1990; Macdonald and Bunton, 1992; Wilkinson, 1994). For the most part the accounts focus on action by individuals and groups or teams of workers within local geographical communities and provide examples of local initiatives attempting to achieve health gain for populations and illustrate how nurses and other healthcare professionals are:

- identifying their clients' health and social needs in areas of high deprivation
- speaking out on behalf of individuals, families, and communities suffering from poverty and deprivation
- fighting for more resources in these areas of need
- identifying poverty as a factor in their caseload profiles
- providing a targeting health and social need commentary for managers and policy-makers.

These exemplars also demonstrate in most cases that community practitioners' activities can change behaviour, practice, the community and the environment. From an inequality perspective their efforts are directed at:

- raising the awareness of social exclusion, poverty and deprivation as an urban and rural issue
- raising the profile of inequalities in health
- assessing health and social needs
- training lay health workers within communities
- helping to increase individuals' self-esteem, coping skills, motivation, knowledge, insight and experience
- providing group work and support for communities
- employing local people
- providing services such as counselling, drop-in centres, support groups, mental health groups, screening clinics for the homeless and those with learning disabilities, parent-craft classes for minority ethnic groups.

The idea of promoting health within the framework of inequalities may, depending on its nature, highlight the epidemiological, psychological, sociological, or concentrate on issues of social policy, research and health promotion. The emphasis on health promotion within inequalities evaluation suggests that it is oriented towards producing a greater understanding of the ways of achieving intersectoral working, community development, equity and a reduction in inequalities in health and social wellbeing. It is clear from these case studies that nurses and healthcare professionals are using well designed more qualitative evaluation methods in such a way that they have demonstrated an improvement in health and social need for those in the lowest socio-economic groups. There is increasing acknowledgement that quantitative methods that meet the criteria of statistical robustness can leave minority and vulnerable voices unheard. The use of qualitative evaluation opens the door to measures of social position that reflect the ways in which people define themselves and the relationships which sustain them. This allows community practitioners to ask people how they are experiencing inequalities in health and their needs. 'Effective practice' and effectiveness should focus on the needs of clients – what they really want and need and how they want it (Lazenbatt and Orr, 2001).

However, while these interventions are encouraging there is a great deal more research to be undertaken to satisfy sound evaluation methods. Recommendations suggest that for nursing to show evidence of quality and the effectiveness of interventions it must do so through more formal evaluation techniques. This requires the development of an evaluative culture that encourages a research evidence-based approach and the application of methods to improve the quality of care as well as the treatments and services that practitioners offer their patients and clients. Most practitioners will not want to become researchers, but they should be able to appreciate the evaluation methods of others and understand how to incorporate evaluation findings into their own professional practice. Evaluation must be used to improve the quality of an intervention and provide evidence of effectiveness, efficiency, equity and cost effectiveness and 'best' practice as well as of the contribution that it is making to improve the health and wellbeing of individuals and groups.

PROMOTING HEALTH AND WELLBEING

In any area of work there will always be a debate about what constitutes 'best' practice. Not every health promoter finds it easy to acknowledge economic and social determinants of health and social need in his or her practice but should realize that poverty and deprivation are determined by a number of complex and often interrelating factors such as:

income and social position	limited education
gender	unemployment or low income
geographical location	lack of social support networks
age	social exclusion
lifestyle	poor housing
disability	sexual orientation
culture and race	

It is increasingly recognized that the experience of inequalities in health and social need reflects the interaction of a number of these factors: people occupy not one but multiple social positions which all bear consequences for health. Research shows that people in disadvantaged groups not only suffer more ill health and die younger, but they are less likely to receive or benefit from health and social care (Benzeval, 1995).

TACKLING INEQUALITIES IN HEALTH AND SOCIAL NEED?

A report by the King's Fund contains an impressive agenda for action (Benzeval et al., 1995; 1997) and suggests four levels of intervention:

1   improving the physical environment
2   addressing social and economic factors
3   reducing barriers to adopting a healthier personal lifestyle
4   improving access to appropriate and effective health and social services.

Margaret Whitehead (1992) provides a detailed review of interventions in various countries and suggests that policy initiatives can influence inequalities in health in four different ways:

1   strengthening individuals
2   strengthening communities
3   improving access to essential facilities and services
4   encouraging macroeconomic and cultural change.

At the first level interventions have been employed to include preventive and screening services as well as strategies to strengthen people such as support networks, stress management education, smoking cessation clinics and counselling of the unemployed to prevent a decline in their physical and mental health. Interventions at this level rely on community nurses, midwives and health visitors to concentrate on maternal and child health. These sorts of strategies, if they are targeted at disadvantaged groups in society, may have a direct effect on inequalities in health by decreasing their prevalence of smoking or increasing their uptake of immunization services. The second level is concerned with how people in disadvantaged areas and communities combine to strengthen their resistance against health hazards. This involves fostering the strengths of families, communities and others from healthcare fields in combination with voluntary and self-help groups to form influential collaborations and partnerships. These can help to inform and influence healthier alliances and conditions for local disadvantaged communities.

The third policy level is about improving access to healthcare and the provision of adequate social services. People need access to adequate housing, clean water, sanitation, secure employment, adequate nutrition and essential health and social care services. Intersectoral collaborations and partnerships are required to impact upon health at this level. Such policies will benefit the health of all the population, however, if they are targeted at disadvantaged groups and communities; they will contribute more to people living in the worst conditions and therefore have a potential to reduce inequalities in health and social need. The final level does not deal directly with inequalities in health but with wider inequalities in society. It is concerned with the distribution of income in wealth between rich and poor in society. Whitehead (1992) further stresses that a person's health cannot be divorced from the social and economic environment in which he/she lives. She identifies as factors of critical importance:

- the physical environment (adequate housing, working conditions and pollution)
- social and economic influences such as income and wealth, levels of unemployment, and the quality of social relationships and social support
- barriers to adopting a healthier lifestyle
- access to appropriate and effective health and social services.

These factors suggest that the distribution of health and ill health in the population reflects a profoundly unequal distribution of resources in society. She relates these to a number of areas of importance which require the inclusion of women, older people and members of minority groups. In addition, she advocates equity in access to healthcare services and calls for improvement in community-based services. We know that it is important for practitioners to actively promote and enhance the quality of life and wellbeing of their patients and clients, not simply by preventing disease but to assess and define parameters of positive health – in other words to understand 'what keeps people healthy' and to strengthen people to take action. Throughout this handbook the words 'health promotion' denote an activity which identifies the factors that may influence health and evaluation of activities related to the promotion of health. These include areas such as the facilitation and promotion of healthy environments, the development and strengthening of personal skills and support mechanisms, the provision of better access to health and social care services, and the encouragement of community participation, and empowerment.

THE EQUITY ISSUE

Because of the differing understandings about health inequalities, several WHO documents have preferred to use the term 'equity'.

Equity in health means that ideally everyone should have a fair opportunity to attain their full health potential and, more pragmatically, that no one should be disadvantaged from achieving his or her potential (WHO, 1985).

In economists' terms, the best use of resources is that which maximizes benefits to society as a whole. Similarly, although a given healthcare intervention might maximize benefits to society as a whole, in doing so it might increase differences in the amount of benefit received by different groups in society – in other words it might actually widen inequalities in health and in the need for and access to care.

For example, if we look at how increased rates of uptake for screening for cervical cancer might reduce mortality rates for society as a whole, it is interesting to note that uptake rates for social classes IV and V are far lower than those in higher social classes. However, if we scrutinize this further we see that, although it is increasing the rate of uptake for society as a whole, it may be increasing differences in the amount of benefit experienced by those belonging to different social classes.

There is a contest of ideas between economic evaluators and healthcare professionals who believe that deprived people should be afforded better access to healthcare in proportion to their greater need. In contrast, economists argue that if equity is the main objective rather than efficiency, then the overall health of the population would be worse. However, such differences apart, both groups have a lot to learn from each other.

On the one hand, health practitioners have taught economists that efficiency cannot be the only criterion in deciding on the best use of resources if this discriminates against the more deprived sections of society. On the other hand, economists have taught health practitioners that if they decide to use up scarce resources on one group of patients these resources are not available to others. Health practitioners therefore need to choose between meeting different health needs, and in the face of scarce resources to prioritize the costs and benefits in a rational and systematic way.

In order to target corrective action, the equitable provision of healthcare must begin with a systematic assessment of the needs of sub-groups and the risks that they face (Lazenbatt, 1999; Lazenbatt et al., 2000a). However, even if healthcare services were distributed between areas in direct proportion to their relative need, that distribution would not automatically result in equal access to healthcare for all social groups. Available resources are not always allocated in the most efficient way to meet the needs of their populations and different social groups may face different barriers to access. Moreover, there are groups of people who have unequal access to services and require health and social care but do not avail themselves of services such as health checks, screening, well-focused care, self-help or support groups.

'HARD-TO-REACH' GROUPS

These groups may have barriers to healthier lifestyles because of finances, geography, language, culture or communication. Communication as a barrier may not simply mean that participants are speaking a different language but it may be that the primary care or clinical teams have failed to communicate effectively. The problem may be deeper in that inequalities exist because the group or individual may not share the professional's views about the importance of healthcare or they may find the service on offer to be inappropriate or even threatening to themselves or their cultural background. Such groups may include:

- ethnic and cultural minorities
- travellers
- homeless people
- those individuals with mental or psychological illness, and learning disabilities
- adolescents
- gay men
- bisexuals
- lesbians
- substance abusers
- prostitutes
- lone parents
- older people.

These barriers include:

- Geographical barriers – facilities may not be easily accessed from rural areas without a car and this leads to disadvantaged groups becoming reliant on public transport which can be expensive, inconvenient and unreliable.
- Cultural barriers – users may have different social and cultural backgrounds from healthcare workers and this can hinder communication and effective care.
- Logistical barriers – people in employment tied to business hours, lone parents with young children, elderly and disabled people, or those who have caring responsibilities may find it difficult to access health services.

Successful interventions must work towards the removal of such barriers by highlighting the need for enhanced accessibility, for example by meeting language needs, training staff to be culturally and communicatively sensitive, and by providing specific clinics and services which are user-sensitive such as outreach clinics, healthy living centres and drop-in centres (Lazenbatt, 1999; Lazenbatt and Hunter, 2000; Lazenbatt and Orr, 2001).

FURTHER READING

Benzeval, M., Judge, K. and Whitehead, M. (1995) *Tackling Inequalities in Health – An Agenda for Action*. London: The King's Fund.
Benzeval, M., Judge, K. and Whitehead, M. (1997) Tackling inequalities in health – an agenda for action. *Sociology of Health and Illness*, 19(1): 127–128.
Benzeval, M. (1998) *Poverty and Public Health – Finally on the Agenda*. London: CPHVA.
Black, D., Morris, J., Smith, C. and Townsend, P. (1980) *Inequalities in Health: Report of a*

Working Group Chaired by Sir Douglas Black. London: Department of Health and Social Security.

Blaxter, M. (1990) Whose fault is it ? People's own conceptions of the reasons for inequalities in health. *Social Science and Medicine*, 44(6): 747–756.

Department of Health (1992) *Health of the Nation: A Strategy for Health in England*. HMSO: London.

Department of Health (2001) *The National Health Inequalities Targets* (www.doh.gov.uk/healthinequalities).

Independent Inquiry into Inequalities in Health (1998) *Independent Inquiry into Inequalities in Health Report* (Acheson Report). London: The Stationery Office.

Lazenbatt, A. (1997) *Targeting Health and Social Need, Volume 1: The Contribution of Nurses, Midwives and Health Visitors*. Belfast: The Stationery Office.

Lazenbatt, A. (1999) *Manual for Evaluation and Effectiveness in Practice, Volume 2*. Belfast: The Stationery Office.

Lazenbatt, A. (2000) Tackling inequalities in health in Northern Ireland. *Community Practitioner*, 73(2): 481–483.

Lazenbatt, A. and Hunter, P. (2000) 'An evaluation of a drop-in centre for working women'. Queen's University of Belfast/Royal College of Nursing, Northern Ireland.

Lazenbatt, A., Sinclair, M., Salmon, S. and Calvert, J. (2001) Telemedicine as a support system to encourage breastfeeding in Northern Ireland: a case study design. *Journal of Telemedicine and Telecare* (in press).

Lazenbatt, A. and Orr, J. (2001) Evaluation and effectiveness in practice. *International Journal of Nursing Practice*, 7(6) (in press).

Lazenbatt, A., McWhirter, L., Bradley, M, and Orr, J. (1999) The role of nursing partnership interventions in improving the health of disadvantaged women. *Journal of Advanced Nursing*, 30 (6), 1280–1288.

Lazenbatt, A., McWhirter, L., Bradley, M. and Orr, J. (2000a) Community nursing achievements in targeting health and social need. *Nursing Times Research*, 5(3), 178–192.

Lazenbatt, A., McWhirter, L., Bradley, M., Orr, J. and Chambers, M. (2000b) Tackling inequalities in health and social wellbeing – evidence of 'good practice' by nurses, midwives and health visitors. *International Journal of Nursing Practice*, 6(2) April: 76–88.

Lazenbatt, A., Lynch, U. and O'Neill, E. (2001) Revealing the hidden 'troubles' in Northern Ireland: the role of Participatory Rapid Appraisal. *Health Education Research* (in press).

Macdonald, G. and Bunton, R. (1992) Health promotion discipline or disciplines. In *Health Promotion Disciplines and Diversity*. London: Routledge.

Secretary of State for Health (2000) *The NHS Plan*, Cmd. 4818–1. London: The Stationery Office.

Whitehead, M. (1987) *The Health Divide*. London: Health Education Council.

Whitehead, M. (1992). The health divide. In Townsend, P., Whitehead, M. and Davidson, N. (eds) *Inequalities in Health and the Health Divide*, second edition. London: Penguin.

Whitehead, M. (1992) Tackling inequalities: a review of policy initiatives. In M. Benzeval, K. Judge and M. Whitehead (eds) *Tackling Inequalities in Health: An Agenda for Action*. London: King's Fund.

Wilkinson, R G. (1994) *Unfair Shares; The Effects of Widening Income Differences on the Welfare of the Young*. London: Barnardo's.

World Bank (1997) *Health Aspects of Environmental Impact Assessment*. Environmental assessment sourcebook update. Washington DC: World Bank.

World Health Organisation (1985) *Targets for Health for All*. Copenhagen: WHO.

CHAPTER 3

EVIDENCE-BASED HEALTHCARE

UNDERSTANDING 'BEST' PRACTICE

There appears to be no international or nationally accepted definition of 'best' practice. However, as Sheldon (1994) suggests, there are a number of desirable attributes which might be taken as evidence of best or effective practice which include:

- Validity   Correctly interpreting available evidence so that when followed valid guidelines lead to improvements in health.
- Replication   Given the same evidence another group produces similar recommendations.
- Reliability   Given the same circumstances another health professional applies them similarly.
- Flexibility   Indicates how patients'/clients' views can be incorporated into the decision-making process.
- Clarity   The use of precise definitions and user-friendly language.
- Dissemination   Spreading the word.

The debate concerning best practice is one that views at one end of a continuum the positivist model which has at its basis the assumption that 'objective' facts can be established, while the other end views a phenomenological model taking the social world as being constructed by human beings. Both ends of the continuum produce research and evaluation strategies such as qualitative and quantitative methodologies that are likewise in opposition. Quantitative measures (Frazer *et al.*, 1995) include methods such as the randomized control trial or quasi-experimental design, and the large-scale survey, while qualitative methods (Secker, 1995) include ethnographies and approaches that seek to interpret and contextualize, such as participant and non-participant observation, unstructured and semi-structured interviews and focus groups and interviews and content analysis. With this continuing debate, many evaluators find it difficult to decide the extent to which the findings from both of these methodologies are compatible or comparable. The reality of the evidence is that evaluators appear to use both techniques.

Hutchinson (1995) argues that there is no clear rationale or structured reasons for selecting methods along the continuum from qualitative to quantitative. He suggests that the choice of method is not always based on a consideration of the appropriateness of the evaluation tool for the particular intervention. The development of evaluation in an applied technical environment has led to the dominant focus on measurable outcomes and the neglect of methodologies for evaluating process and for transferring experience from one intervention to another. Moreover, if according to Bunton *et al.* (1994), we adopt rigorous experimental methodological principles and measures of effectiveness then a large number of studies are inconclusive. There are few interventions to promote health that show unequivocal evidence of reducing morbidity and mortality, but this may be partly due to the fact that there is a paucity of evaluation that takes account of these measures. Wadsworth (1997) states that one of the major problems in this area has been the sterile epistemological arguments between evaluators favouring quantitative and qualitative methods, between phenomenological and positivist social scientists and between those who are advocates of the random controlled trial (RCT) to the exclusion of evaluations of process and delivery of novel prevention programmes. His work exemplifies the need to be methodologically eclectic and not become bound by epistemological constraints if we are to develop new interventions and demonstrate their effectiveness.

MOVE TO EVIDENCE-BASED HEALTHCARE

Evidence-based healthcare is defined as the conscientious, explicit, and judicious use of current best practice in making decisions about the care of patients and treatment of individuals. The practice of evidence-based healthcare means integrating individual clinical expertise with best available evidence from systematic research (Sackett, 1996). The ideas behind evidence-based healthcare have provoked much debate, including challenges to the assertion that 80% of medical treatments are of unproven value. However, most of the systematic reviews include only studies that are based on experimental design (testing theories and causality) which is traditionally seen as the only valid way to evaluate treatments and services. Claims have been made that effectiveness from health visiting, health promotion, alternative therapies, community health and other community services are untestable in these terms, and a danger exists that the impact of evidence-based healthcare may become undermined if a practical solution to untestability is not found.

Researchers and practitioners have long been concerned with designing appropriate evaluation and effectiveness studies. However, very little effort has been spent on either assessing the quality of the research design or assessing the effectiveness through literature reviews. The movement towards establishing evidence for clinical effectiveness has led to the establishment of a number of centres specializing in mechanisms for measuring effective outcomes. The Cochrane Collaborating Centres and others have established scientific rigour in their quest to prepare and disseminate systematic reviews on the effects of healthcare interventions. The Cochrane Library was initially set up to provide systematic reviews of maternity services and now covers research on most areas of healthcare which has involved the development of a hierarchy of evidence, largely based on quantitative measures with emphasis on randomized control trials and 'hard' scientific evidence. The Cochrane Library (www.cochrane.co.uk/info) now contains:

- the Cochrane Database of Systematic Reviews (CDSR)
- the York Database of Abstracts of Reviews of Effectiveness (DARE)
- the Cochrane Pregnancy and Childbirth Database
- the Cochrane Controlled Trials Register (CCTR)
- the Cochrane Review methodology Database (CRMD).

Another excellent source of systematically reviewed and appraised research is *Clinical Evidence* which is available as a book or on the internet. It is updated and expanded every six months and is published by the British Medical Journal (BMJ) publishing group (www.clinical evidence.org). The work of the NHS Centre for Reviews and Dissemination (CRD), University of York, and the Social Science Research Unit, Institute of Education (University of London) also pose significant challenges to all those who are engaged in health-promoting interventions to improve the quality of life of individuals and provide equity of services. The CRD produces effectiveness bulletins which address a variety of topics and full details of all CRD publications can be found on the centre's website (www.york.ac.uk/inst/crd).

Current systematic reviews of published material and meta-analysis of the data are based on a hierarchy of evidence (Sheldon, 1994), with or without the cost-effectiveness element. As Figure 3.1 demonstrates the RCT has been seen as the true experimental design or 'gold standard' for quantitative evaluative research as it can eliminate confounding variables. However, this is only the case if the RCT is well designed and carried out. A well-conducted quasi-experimental design without the benefit of randomization to experimental and control groups may provide better 'evidence' of effect than a poor RCT. Indeed, much published material on effectiveness (Nutbeam and Wise, 1996) has focused on outcome rather than research design.

Even where reviews have combined assessment of methodology with effectiveness, the implications for promoting health within interventions and their impact on health status is unclear (Nuffield Institute for Health, 1993), or limited (Garcia, 1994). Recently the term 'knowledge-based practice' has been used by Graham Hart and his colleagues

---

1   Intervention studies
   1a Randomized control trial (RCT)
   1b Controlled trial (non-randomized)
   1c Quasi-experimental design (QED)

2   Observational studies
   2a Cohort (prospective) study
   2b Case-control (respective) study
   2c 'Before' and 'after' studies (no controls)
   2d Descriptive studies: reports on clinical or practitioner
      experience – surveys

Figure 3.1   A research evidence hierarchy. Adapted from Sheldon (1994)

in the MRC Medical Sociology Unit to indicate that what constitutes evidence may include qualitative data and analyses and that a single methodology such as an RCT is not always feasible or indeed desirable in every evaluation. The recent demand for evidence-based medicine has led to the commissioning of a variety of meta-analyses of the literature with a view to identifying the most effective strategies for achieving health gain and at the same time curtailing the escalating costs of healthcare provision. Others have proposed that similar principles need to be applied to decision-making in policy formulation (evidence-based policy-making).

The new requirements of clinical governance are also a challenge for everyone working in the NHS. The UK government's document, *A First Class Service* (1998), defines clinical governance as 'a framework through which NHS organisations are accountable for the quality of clinical care'. If the quality of healthcare is to be improved, existing knowledge about effective clinical and organizational practice must be applied and new information to monitor and evaluate care must be generated and interpreted. Clinical governance aims to integrate these various systems for quality improvement and professional development and to ensure that everyone in the practice team becomes involved. Indeed, an underlying challenge for clinical governance in primary and community care is to move away from professional development based on unidisciplinary education towards multidisciplinary, team-based learning and practice. According to Pringle (2000) clinical governance represents a new formulation of age-old activities:

1   Clinical governance is intended to improve standards of care and at the same time to protect the public from unacceptable care.
2   The move from continuing medical education for nurses and doctors to continuing professional development for the whole primary care team presents new challenges for multidisciplinary learning and performance monitoring.
3   To deal with poor performance, clinical governance leaders will need skills to assess the nature of the problem, educational resources to deal with it, and managerial resources to facilitate the process.
4   Participation in the activities of clinical governance will be an essential feature of revalidation.

Previously, the Royal College of Nursing established a range of quality improvement systems in the 1980s, including the practitioner-led dynamic standard setting system (Morrell *et al.*, 1997), and mechanisms for clinical supervision and reflective practice (RCN, 1998). The Royal College of General Practitioners has also developed assessment mechanisms for general practitioners linked to objective national standards (RCGP, 1999). Within individual general practices and primary care teams, all staff will have a role in obtaining and using information for clinical governance whether for maintaining chronic disease registers, promoting evidence-based practice, improving the organiza-tion of services, or reporting on the outcomes of care. In primary care groups and trusts, there will be greater emphasis on improving the health of the population and this will require the collection and aggregation of information across practices to assess health needs and health impacts, reduce inequalities, and monitor the quality of care in comparison to agreed standards.

Health impact assessment (HIA) has emerged to identify those activities and policies likely to have major impacts on the health of a population. Lock (2000) states that HIA is based on a broad holistic model of health, which proposes that economic, political, social, psychological, and environmental factors determine population health. As it is now widely accepted that the determinants of health inequalities lie outside the health sector, the greatest scope for improving the public's health requires the growth of new policies beyond this sector. As we know, building healthy public policy was a key component of the Ottawa Charter for Health Promotion (WHO, 1986) so therefore the basic concepts of health impact assessment are not new. According to Lock (2000), health impact assessment

1   is a structured method for assessing and improving the health consequences of projects and policies in the health and non-health sector
2   is a multidisciplinary process combining a range of qualitative and quantitative evidence in a decision-making framework
3   includes national policy appraisal, local urban planning, transport, and water and agricultural projects
4   includes benefits such as improved inter-agency collaboration and public participation
5   has limitations including a lack of agreed methods and gaps in the evidence base for health impacts.

Using this broad holistic model of health means that almost any area of public policy can have health impacts. HIA builds on and collates methods familiar to those working in public health and includes policy appraisal, health collaboration and advocacy, community development, evaluation tools, and evidence-based healthcare. It is therefore an eclectic combination of methods whose aim is to assess the health consequences to a population of a policy, project, or programme that does not necessarily have health as its primary objective (Scott Samuel, 1997; 1998). Moreover, it is a multidisciplinary process within which a range of evidence about the health effects of a proposal is considered in a structured framework. It takes into account the opinions and expectations of those who may be affected by a proposed policy such as policy-makers, organizations, practitioners, patients, and communities.

In 1995, the Department of Health published a discussion document, *Policy Appraisal and Health*, which investigated the importance of public policy as a determinant of health (DoH, 1995). *The Independent Inquiry into Inequalities and Health* (Acheson, 1998) also proposed health impact assessment as a means of identifying and addressing the needs of vulnerable groups in health inequalities impact assessment. Both proposed a framework for assessing health impacts based on economic appraisal methods that had originally been designed to assess health services rather than social policy. HIA methods all emphasize the importance of: focusing on equitable outcomes; explicitly targeting disadvantaged groups; enabling the full participation of those likely to be affected by the policy or project; and using a combination of qualitative as well as quantitative methods of inquiry.

Health impact assessment aims to influence the decision-making process in an open, structured way. To do this it has to acknowledge that assessing and ranking evidence is not a wholly objective process and involves a series of value and more subjective judgments. Political imperatives are likely to affect the outcome. The balance between objective evidence and subjective opinion should be explicitly recognized in reports of assessments. As stated previously, in evidence-based medicine there is a weighted hierarchy of epidemiological evidence, with randomized controlled trials at the top. Obviously this is not useful in assessments where evidence comes from a range of quantitative and qualitative sources.

There is a need to develop a new framework for gathering, interpreting, and prioritizing evidence from different origins for evidence-based policy-making. It must be argued that health-promoting interventions are qualitatively different from medical interventions (Tones and Tilford, 1994; Macdonald, 1996; Scott Samuel, 1998). Macdonald suggests that if the double-blind trial is the jewel in the crown of the RCT, then, by contrast double illumination should constitute the goal of health-promoting evaluation. Process evaluation is essential in order to ascertain the adequacy of programme delivery and illuminative evaluation is necessary to understand what has happened from the perspective of different stakeholders and to provide sufficient information to improve the programme both developmentally and summatively.

INTERVENTIONS TO REDUCE INEQUALITIES IN HEALTH

Whitehead *et al.* (2000) stress that although there is increasing political commitment to tackle inequalities in health, there is a growing awareness that the effectiveness of many of the broader interventions has not been evaluated as in many cases the tools and methodologies to do so are underdeveloped. Therefore the current knowledge on the efficacy of interventions to reduce inequalities in health and social need is extremely scarce. Most interventions have been directed at the individual level and have involved the provision of information and support. The effectiveness of most interventions has not been rigorously evaluated and the outcome measures used, while worthwhile in themselves, are often difficult to relate to the outcomes commonly used in inequalities research literature. Interventions designed to improve the public health in general (for example, mass smoking cessation programmes) have tended to benefit the better off groups more, both because the latter are more likely to be able to respond to such interventions, and because they may benefit more from the behavioural change once made (Macintyre, 1997). There is thus a paradox that the deprivation model now regarded as inappropriate by many researchers may be more feasible and effective as an underlying principle for practical interventions than a linear gradient model.

Although the systematic reviews (Arblaster *et al.*, 1995; Gepkens and Gunning-Schepers, 1995) show that some interventions have short-term benefits for the deprived individuals or communities, it is harder to demonstrate long-term effectiveness in reducing inequalities in health. One difficulty is the insistence of trying to subject such interventions to the standards of a rigorous research design, such as the randomized control trial, and another is the long time span which may be necessary to demonstrate any reduction in inequalities, which may take years or even generations. A commitment to evidence-based healthcare or 'best' practice means a commitment to planning and evaluation: planning to include the needs of the target group and to employ the best of current knowledge as to how to meet these needs; evaluation to find out the effectiveness of the intervention, who has benefited and who has not. This is important as practitioners, policy-makers and fund-holders naturally wish to concentrate resources on programme areas and approaches which are demonstrably effective or 'evidence-based' interventions and which link more closely to need. In the field of health promotion itself it is estimated that no more than 15% of current medical and surgical interventions are directly evidence-based and as few as 5% have been subjected to rigorous evaluations (Macdonald, 1996).

THE NEED FOR EVIDENCE-BASED INTERVENTIONS: INTERNATIONAL EVIDENCE – SYSTEMATIC REVIEWS

Reviews of inequalities in health and social need

Within the area of inequalities in health, evidence of 'best' practice has been gathered from three sources, all suggesting that certain features characterize the successful intervention. The governments in the Netherlands, the UK and Northern Ireland have all commissioned reviews of the literature in search of evaluated possibilities to reduce health inequalities. This discussion will focus on some of the similarities and some of the differences between the three reviews and the consequences for further research.

Review methodology

The three studies covered different time periods with clearly different aims.

The Dutch review, 'Interventions to reduce socio-economic health differences' (Gepkens and Gunning-Schepers, 1995), was the final project of a five-year research programme commissioned by the government between 1989 and 1994. The project was asked to give an overview of examples of interventions that have been implemented and evaluated, aimed at either reducing inequalities or variations in health or improving the health of the lowest socio-economic groups. It included as many interventions done at local level as possible, even though they were often not formally published and are reported only in the so-called 'grey' literature. The Dutch review scanned papers published during 1966–1993 and 98 interventions were identified using the following dimensions:

- target population
- intended effects of the intervention
- the type of intervention method used
- the methods of evaluation
- the actual effects.

The UK systematic review, 'Systemic review of the effectiveness of health service interventions aimed at reducing inequalities in health' (Arblaster et al., 1995) carried out by the NHS Centre for Reviews and Dissemination of York University was commissioned by the Department of Health for its *Variations in Health* report (Department of Health, 1995a) as part of the Health of the Nation initiative. Its aim was to identify interventions which the NHS alone or in collaboration with other agencies could use to improve the health of people from lower socio-economic groups or ethnic minority groups or to reduce differences in health status. The methodological criteria for inclusion were more rigorous than the Dutch or Northern Ireland review. It included only interventions with an experimental design (those involving before and after studies with or without controls, randomized and non-randomized). The UK review systematically reviewed the interventions from 1966 to 1994. Studies were included if they assessed health promotion interventions designed to reduce inequalities in health or improve the health of disadvantaged groups and could be carried out by a health service alone or in collaboration with other agencies. Only studies evaluating interventions using an experimental design were included. A total of 122 were identified and over 30 reviews were included.

The Northern Ireland review, the Targeting Health and Social Need (THSN) Project, was entitled *The Contribution of Nurses, Midwives and Health Visitors to Inequalities in Health* (Lazenbatt, 1997) (Lazenbatt *et al.*, 1999). This was a four-year research programme commissioned by the Northern Ireland government between 1995 and 1999. The project assessed the contribution that nurses, midwives and health visitors were making to interventions which have been implemented and evaluated, aimed at either reducing inequalities or improving the health and social need of those living in poverty or deprived areas or those socially excluded from society. Again it included as many interventions done at local level as possible, even though they were often not formally published and are reported only in the so-called 'grey' literature. It also included interventions with an experimental design (those involving before and after studies with or without controls, randomized and non-randomized). A total of 392 interventions were reviewed and identified by a survey questionnaire using the following selection criteria:

- intervention study
- inequalities groupings such as geographical variations, material deprivation
- areas or groups with a need, vulnerable groups, inter-agency working/lay people
- evaluation and immediate, intermediate or long-term outcomes.

Findings

The Dutch, UK and Northern Ireland reviews identified between 98 and 392 interventions each, of which only 22 were common to all. However, many of the interventions identified by the Northern Ireland and Dutch teams did not meet the rigorous inclusion criteria of the York study (many of which came from the USA). The characteristics of success were similar in all reviews. Within the grey literature many of the projects discussed included the work of nurses, health visitors and midwives working at a local level. The topics covered varied from well women clinics to prevention of domestic violence with emphasis on the empowerment of individuals and communities. Many of the interventions took intermediate endpoints, e.g. increased knowledge, positive changes in attitude or changing behaviour.

All three reviews reflect a very creative and active health promotion field in which innovative approaches are tried, described and sometimes formally evaluated. However, these positive conclusions are overshadowed by the fact that none of the reviews offers a clear basis upon which to build a policy to reduce inequalities in health that is likely to be effective in the short term. The studies were predominantly small-scale, using personal health education or attempting to improve access to healthcare. Many of the studies reported did not measure the effect of the intervention in terms of a reduction of group health differences. From these reviews, do we know if these interventions are more effective in higher socio-economic groups? Indeed, the interventions may improve the health in the lowest groups but do not guarantee a reduction in health differences.

However, Whitehead *et al.* (2000) conclude that while randomized control trials involving individuals are rarely possible (we could never control the numerous extraneous variables or confounding variables in the real world situation), there are circumstances when community intervention trials may be feasible and when the basic rules of the classic study designs could be employed (they are likely to be difficult to design, costly and complicated). The nature of true experimental design depends on random allocation. Without random allocation there can be no guarantee that any observable effects are due to the intervention. Unfortunately random allocation of individuals to experimental and control groups on anything other than a relatively small scale is expensive and problematic. Even if possible, the artificiality of the situation can minimize the possibilities of generalizing the results to 'normal' populations. It is, of course, easier to allocate naturalistic units such as schools or worksites to experimental and comparative conditions. In fact, in community-wide programmes it is all but impossible to ensure that there is no 'leakage' from experimental to control group (Nutbeam and Wise, 1996).

The majority of literature from specialist health promotion sources advocates an economic, individual, social and environmental perspective in evaluation and a battery of data collecting and investigative methodologies (Tones and Tilford, 1994; Macdonald, 1996). These authors suggest that it is often difficult to attribute cause and effect from such evaluations and a more 'pluralistic' approach to evaluation is needed, which will incorporate qualitative and quantitative methods. In conclusion, the most important contribution of these reviews is that they bring together a wide variety of creative ideas. Even though some of the interventions were not scientifically evaluated, their insights might allow future programmes to become so. From the reviews a list of characteristics of successful interventions aimed at proving the health of disadvantaged groups has been developed. Arblaster *et al.* (1995) identify ten characteristics of success (Table 3.1) while eight characteristics of success are highlighted in the Dutch and Northern Irish reviews (Table 3.2).

CHARACTERISTICS OF 'QUALITY INTERVENTIONS'

Synthesis of the findings shown in Tables 3.1 and 3.2 produces a list of characteristics which suggest a 'quality intervention' more likely to impact upon health and social need inequalities. These characteristics are listed at the beginning of the next chapter and then each is illustrated by case studies of quality interventions.

Table 3.1 Characteristics of successful interventions aimed at improving the health of disadvantaged groups, UK systematic review

The points summarized below are the results of reviews which assessed the success of interventions and identified the characteristics which have demonstrated success at improving the health of disadvantaged groups.

1   *Intensive approaches*   Vigorous or intensive approaches have been shown to improve the identification and subsequent effective treatment of individuals, particularly those from deprived populations.

2   *Community commitment*   A number of reviews emphasized the importance of ensuring the community in which the intervention was taking place supported the intervention.

3   *Multidisciplinary approaches*   Here a number of agencies are involved to facilitate the adoption of different strategies, the development of improved information systems and provide more resources.

4   *Multifaceted interventions*   Several successful programmes employed a combination of interventions to improve the health of deprived populations, e.g. a combination of a structured intervention, flexibly delivered and directed by both the client and the professional.

5   *Settings*   Interventions in a variety of settings have been shown to be effective, e.g. involving home visiting.

6   *Prior needs assessment to inform intervention design*   Some studies reported a form of needs assessment of the target group to allow tailoring of the intervention.

7   *Ensuring interventions are culturally appropriate*   Interventions showed sensitivity to the cultural needs of the target group.

8   *Importance of the agent delivering the intervention*   Several successful interventions were carried out by non-professionals, volunteers, often recruited from the target population and trained to perform a task.

9   *Training those delivering the intervention*   A number of reviews have highlighted the importance of training.

10   *Support materials*   This involved using educational materials such as booklets and videos.

Source: Arblaster et al., (1995)

Table 3.2 Characteristics of successful interventions aimed at targeting health and social need in Holland and Northern Ireland

The points summarized below are the results of reviews in Holland and Northern Ireland which assessed the success of interventions and identified the characteristics which demonstrated success in targeting health and social need or reducing socio-economic health differences.

1   *Holistic view of health and social need*   These interventions encompasss the 'whole person' and use the biopsychosocial and environmental model of health.

2   *Health alliances and inter-agency working*   Statutory, community and voluntary groups work together to promote health and raise issues such as inequalities in health.

3   *Empowerment*   This allows the individual/community to take control of their health and social needs.

4   *Research-based approach*   These interventions are concerned with generating new knowledge, theoretical models and evidence of success.

5   *Multidisciplinary working*   Here teams of professionals promote health by collaborative working within supportive networks.

6   *Needs assessment*   This involves profiling to obtain community health needs, population views of health and to identify gaps in service delivery.

7   *Community development*   Partnerships and networks for communities are provided to set priorities, make decisions, plan strategies and implement them to achieve better health.

8   *Audit and evaluation in practice*   Here systematic methods are used for assessing, judging, guiding and improving interventions.

Source: Gepkens and Gunning-Schepers (1995); Lazenbatt (1997)

FURTHER READING

Acheson, D. (1998) *Independent Inquiry into Inequalities in Health*. London: Stationery Office.

Arblaster, L., Lambert, M., Entwhistle, M., Fullerton, D., Sheldon, T. and Watt, I. A. (1995) Systematic review of the effectiveness of health service interventions aimed at reducing inequalities in health. *Journal of Health Services Research and Policy*, 1(2): 93–103.

Bunton, R., Burrows, R., Gillen, K. and Muncer, S. (1994) *Interventions to Promote Health in Economically Deprived Areas: A Critical Review of the Literature – 1994*. A Report to the Northern Regional Health Authority, York.

Department of Health (1995a) *Variations in Health. What can the Department of Health and the National Health Service do?* London: Department of Health.

Department of Health (1995b) *Policy Appraisal and Health*. London: Department of Health.

Frazer, E. (1995) Evaluating health promotion – doing it by numbers. *Health Education Journal*, 54(2): 214–225.

Garcia, J. (1994) *Improving Infant Health: A Literature Review*. Health Education Authority: London.

Gepkens, A. and Gunning-Schepers, L.J. (1995) Reviews of interventions to reduce social inequalities in health: research and policy implications. *Health Education Journal*, 55: 226–238.

Hutchinson, A. (1995) Clinical effectiveness – What are the issues? *Report of a Workshop on Clinical Effectiveness*. York: NHS Centre for Reviews and Dissemination, University of York.

Lazenbatt, A. (1997) *Targeting Health and Social Need, Volume 1: The Contribution of Nurses, Midwives and Health Visitors*. Belfast: The Stationery Office.

Lazenbatt, A. (2000) Tackling inequalities in health in Northern Ireland. *Community Practitioner*, 73(2): 481–483.

Lazenbatt, A. and Hunter, P. (2000) 'An evaluation of a drop-in centre for working women'. Queen's University of Belfast/Royal College of Nursing, Northern Ireland.

Lazenbatt, A. and Orr, J. (2001) Evaluation and effectiveness in practice. *International Journal of Nursing Practice*, 7(6) (in press).

Lazenbatt, A., McWhirter, L., Bradley, M. and Orr, J. (1999) The role of nursing partnership interventions in improving the health of disadvantaged women. *Journal of Advanced Nursing*, 30(6), 1280–1288.

Lazenbatt, A., McWhirter, L., Bradley, M. and Orr, J. (2000a) Community nursing achievements in targeting health and social need. *Nursing Times Research*, 5(3): 178–192.

Lazenbatt, A., McWhirter, L., Bradley, M., Orr, J. and Chambers, M. (2000b) Tackling inequalities in health and social wellbeing – evidence of 'good practice' by nurses, midwives and health visitors. *International Journal of Nursing Practice*, 6(2) April: 76–88.

Lazenbatt, A., Sinclair, M., Salmon, S. and Calvert, J. (2001a) Telemedicine as a support system to encourage breastfeeding in Northern Ireland: a case study design. *Journal of Telemedicine and Telecare* (in press).

Lazenbatt, A., Lynch, U. and O'Neill, E. (2001b) Revealing the hidden 'troubles' in Northern Ireland: the role of Participatory Rapid Appraisal. *Health Education Research* (in press).

Lock, K. (2000) Health Impact Assessment. *British Medical Journal*, 320: 1395–1398.

Macdonald, G. (1996) Where next for evaluation? *Health Promotion International*, 11: 34–43.

Macintyre, S. (1997) The Black Report and Beyond: what are the issues? *Social Science and Medicine*, 44(6): 723–746.

Morrell, C., Harvey, G. and Kitson, A. (1997) Practitioner based quality improvement: a review of the RCN's dynamic standard setting system. *Quality in Health Care*, 6: 9–34.

Nuffield Institute for Health (1993) *Effective Health Care 6*. York: University of Leeds.

Nutbeam, D. and Wise, M. (1996) Planning for health for all: international experience in setting health goals and targets. *Health Promotion International*, 11(3): 219–226.

Pringle, M. (2000) Clinical governance in primary care. *British Medical Journal*, 321: 737–740.

Rathwell, T. (1992) Realities of HFA 2000. *Social Science and Medicine*, 35(4): 541–547.

Royal College of Nursing (1998) *Guidance for Nurses on Clinical Governance*. London: RCN.

Royal College of General Practitioners (1999) *Criteria for Membership by Assessment of Performance*. London: RCGP.

Royal College of General Practitioners (1999) *Criteria for Fellowship by Assessment*. London: RCGP.

Sackett, D. (1996) Evidence-based medicine: what it is and what it isn't. *British Medical Journal*, 312: 71–72.

Sackett, D.L. (1996) *Evidence-based Medicine: How to Practice and Teach EBM*. London: Churchill Livingstone.

Scott Samuel, A. (1997) Assessing how public policy impacts on health. *Healthlines*, 47: 15–17.

Scott Samuel, A. (1998) Health impact assessment theory into practice. *Journal of Epidemiology and Community Health*, 52: 704–705.

Secker, J. (1995) Qualitative methods in health promotion research: some criteria for quality. *Health Education Journal*, 54(1): 74–87.

Secretary of State for Health (1999) *Saving Lives: Our Healthier Nation*. London: Stationery Office.

Sheldon, T. (1994) *Report of a Workshop on Clinical Effectiveness*. York: NHS Centre for Reviews and Dissemination, University of York.

Tones, K. and Tilford, S. (1994) *Health Education – Effectiveness, Efficiency and Equity*. London: Chapman and Hall.

Wadsworth, M. (1997) Health inequalities in the life course perspective. *Social Science and Medicine*, 44(6): 859–869.

Whitehead, M., Diderichsen, F. and Burstrom, B. (2000) Researching the impact of public policy on inequalities in health. In Graham, H. (ed.) *Understanding Health Inequalities*. Buckingham: Open University Press.

World Bank (1997) *Health Aspects of Environmental Impact Assessment*. Environmental assessment sourcebook update. Washington DC: World Bank.

World Health Organisation (1986) *The Ottawa Charter: Principles for Health Promotion*. Copenhagen: WHO regional office for Europe.

CHAPTER 4

EFFECTIVENESS AND EVALUATION IN PRACTICE – CASE STUDIES

The following case study examples demonstrate how nurses and healthcare professionals are making efforts to change behaviour, practice, the community and the environment. Each example illustrates one of the eight quality criteria cited in the previous chapter:

- Holistic view of health
- Health alliances/multidisciplinary working
- Needs assessment
- Research-based approach
- Intensive/multifaceted approach
- Audit/evaluation
- Cultural needs
- Importance of the setting, delivery agent and training
- Community development
- Empowerment

In many cases professional boundaries and statutory organizations have been opened up, have been made more flexible and have developed more co-operative negotiated approaches to areas of health and social need. Issues such as openness, structure, equity and accessibility have been addressed. The approaches empower patients and clients to seek active involvement in various aspects of health promotion. As is evidenced by the case studies, practitioners are bringing together skills in articulating health and social need problems, sustaining alliances and evaluating services, recognizing the benefits of informed practice and care. They are offering flexible services that are wide-ranging and socially orientated and building stronger working teams. They include community health needs assessment based on profiles, development of health promotion programmes and health alliances, community initiatives, specialist services and community-based services across GP and inter-agency boundaries. The list below offers examples of the applications from the case studies:

- a wide range of the delivery service areas such as community, primary healthcare, hospital, voluntary sector
- a wide range of different roles undertaken by nurses, midwives and health visitors in collaboration with other professions and client groups

- illustrations of several types of nursing practice – clinical, managerial, facilitator, leadership roles, voluntary capacity, education and research
- a range of new service developments such as major funding extensions, changes to service, and existing practice well done.

In general, the 'best practice' as illustrated in these examples were directed at influencing community and individual behaviour by means of health education, promotion, screening, audit, needs assessment and research. Nurses and healthcare professionals were seen as active members of health alliances and were eager to embrace their roles as part of multidisciplinary teams. The extent of collaboration between the different disciplines and professions was clear and produced examples of positive and favourable outcomes for patients and clients. In some cases intersectoral working and networking provided a means for communicating competencies and transferable skills.

1   HOLISTIC VIEW OF HEALTH
A Well Woman Centre

Most of the interventions explored in some depth viewed health and social need within a holistic model. The 'whole' person has many parts, i.e. the physical, the spiritual, the emotional, the mental, the social. Environmental aspects of health were also included such as adequate housing, sanitation, employment. Also looking beyond the client themselves several interventions illustrated that it is important to promote the health of carers who are often at risk of a breakdown in their health as a result of the additional work and stress of caring for the patient. The following case study illustrates that there are a number of ways in which health professionals can enhance the health and wellbeing of people and communities.

Targeting health and social need

The Well Woman Centre is based in a relatively conservative city with one of the highest levels of poverty and unemployment in Europe. The common perception of a woman's group as being radically feminist had precluded many vulnerable women seeking the support they needed to cope with the stress and health problems associated with living and bringing up a family in poverty. Through the somewhat fragmented network of women's groups in the area, there was a swell of support for a place for women to feel comfortable and confident to discuss, share and tackle their health needs as women on their own terms. The idea of a Well Woman Centre seemed to transcend other political and ideological divisions among existing women's groups and was a concept to which all women could relate. The centre's programmes are holistic, non-clinical and non-discriminatory, and for women and run by women.

Between 180 and 200 women per week attend the centre and it receives between 550 and 600 telephone queries per month. The importance of user participation in defining local health and social problems is recognized by the policy-makers, as is the need for a multidisciplinary and community development approach. The centre recognizes inequalities in health around issues such as gender and social class. The priority has been actively to include the most vulnerable and isolated women in terms of their position in society but also to reach women who either are or perceive themselves to be geographically isolated both from services and centres of decision-making.

Aims and objectives

The Well Woman Centre is based on a participatory, non-hierarchical structure with the philosophy that women and health must be treated holistically. The centre aims not only to provide alternative and effective woman-centred services but also to reach out to women who feel alienated by the medical system and to those professionals whose work affects women's health, in order to establish a more positive and equal relationship. The centre undertakes to:

- provide women with the choice of a comprehensive and assessable woman-centred service in a relaxed non-clinical atmosphere run by women for women – which encompasses the whole range of women's health issues
- provide an alternative service to women who may, because of their age, culture, sexuality, class, marital status or racial origin, be feeling alienated or disempowered by the prevailing medical system
- promote a non-medical view of mental health issues and to challenge the current medicalization of mental and physical ill health
- seek more effective ways of meeting women's health needs by listening to women and encouraging them to develop their own knowledge and expertise through the use of support and community development
- develop constructive and positive relationships with medical, nursing, social work and voluntary services which facilitate the establishment of referral, information and mutual support systems allowing women to be treated as equal partners
- recognize and welcome the contribution that alternative therapies, with their focus of holistic health and on the individual woman, can make to a woman-centred service
- promote health education for women by liaison with existing health education services and, where appropriate, development of its own health education campaigns, to raise public consciousness about women's health issues, levels of service provision and environmental issues
- provide on-going training for professionals, volunteers and women who are interested in developing their own skills and knowledge of women's healthcare.

How the centre works

The project offers two counselling services, generic and cancer. The generic team deal with a broad range of issues from sexual abuse, relationship difficulties to eating disorders, and has seven counsellors all of whom have a qualification in counselling. There are 11 counsellors on the cancer counselling service. This service is solely for those who have been given a diagnosis of cancer.

Clinics

The centre runs four clinical services:

- Menopause Clinic – a joint project between the Well Woman Centre and the Community Trust
- Weekly Breast Examination Clinic – run by a local health visitor
- Cervical Smear and Breast Examination Service – a joint venture between the Well Woman Centre and Action Cancer
- Cholesterol and Blood Pressure Testing Service – run by the Well Woman Centre and the Chest, Heart and Stroke Association.

Support Services

The centre runs ten groups each of which is facilitated by a woman who has lived through the issue and a trained medical practitioner therapist. The groups are a menopause group, postnatal depression therapy group, premenstrual tension group, sexual abuse survivors' group, cancer group, breastfeeding group, hysterectomy group, eating disorders therapy group, child loss group, information group, and a dyslexia group.

Health Promotion

The centre runs a series of courses and classes and takes part in events with the aim of promoting good health. All classes are facilitated by qualified staff from various multi-professional backgrounds and include classes such as healthy eating/wholefood cookery, antenatal /parentcraft, know your own body, getting better, self-confidence/ self-esteem building and empowerment, and breastfeeding awareness.

Complementary therapies

The centre teaches and provides the following range of therapies including reflexology, aromatherapy, homeopathy, yoga, and Bach flower remedies.

Evaluation

In-house reviews and audits are undertaken for all the support groups and courses. Funding has been generated to allow a more extensive evaluation of all the services.

Immediate successful outcomes

The centre has been successful in:

- improving the quality of life and wellbeing of women and communities
- providing a specialized service
- engaging the community with professionals links
- generating health interest within the community at neighbourhood level
- promoting lifestyle issues
- campaigning for improvements in care
- securing major funding for the future.

It has also identified the following problems:

- initial lack of resources
- general problems of individuals working within a group situation
- problems of dealing with grief when a client dies in a support group
- travelling and transport difficulties for the clients' group.

Characteristics of best practice in the Well Woman Centre

- an agreed holistic philosophy
- motivated, committed and skilled multidisciplinary staff
- decisions based on needs assessment
- planned approach
- working in partnerships and health alliances
- realistic aims
- overcoming resistance
- use of effective methods
- consumer involvement
- improving the health and quality of life of women in the local community
- cross-community working
- disseminating results
- monitoring and evaluation
- research-based approach
- future funding.

2   HEALTH ALLIANCES AND INTER-AGENCY WORKING

Childhood Accident Prevention Project

Community groups and voluntary organizations working together with the statutory services are promoting health and raising the issues concerned with inequalities. If health promotion is to become effective the idea of community participation must be put into practice, so the voluntary sector, community groups and similar social networks have a central part to play and may be an important resource in the process of enabling people to increase control over or improve their health and social wellbeing. The interventions show voluntary organizations or management leading the development of new services, clinics and counselling services; they also obtain the co-operation of other health professionals, agencies and authorities and voluntary organizations in jointly planning and delivering the service. 'Best practice' involves nurses collaborating with others and allowing themselves to be inventive in identifying changed healthcare practice in meeting targeted health and social needs.

Targeting health and need

The Childhood Accident Prevention Programme (CAPP) is an innovative programme developed to address the high incidence of childhood accidents. It follows the UK Government in its strategy document, *Health of the Nation*, which identified a reduction in the death rate among children under the age of 15 years by at least 33% as one of its key targets. The project has acted upon the principles of addressing the needs of an area with intrinsic rather than extrinsic approaches. In order to facilitate an accident prevention policy the process was initiated through the development of health alliances and an inter-agency group to pool resources. This group consisted of members from both voluntary and statutory agencies. The inter-agency group meet monthly to define targets, provide expertise and guidance, and support a core accident prevention team.

Aims and objectives

The aims and objectives of the programme are to:

- communicate with the community through health alliances and inter-agency working
- raise awareness of accident prevention in a community setting
- provide a forum for the identification of local needs in relation to accidents and their prevention
- transfer knowledge, new skills, information and support to local activities
- initiate intervention programmes within a broad-based approach to meet the needs of the targeted groups
- increase awareness of accident risk and stimulate an increased involvement in accident prevention.

Target groups

The main target group were children and young people. This also included those involved with children such as mother and toddler groups, crèches, nurseries, schools, teachers, grandparents, foster parents, community groups, libraries, scouts, brownies, guides etc.

Development of the accident prevention programme

Information packs

In recognizing the needs of the community and the issues pertinent to that area, information packs were developed to assist community groups in fostering an awareness of accident prevention. Initially a series of ten information packs were developed. It was hoped that the packs would provide a structure to the education process and facilitate the community in identifying their own needs in relation to accident prevention. The information pack had three sections: one providing the facilitator with current information on the specific accident, one on group work, and one on guidelines on how to establish a productive workshop environment and details which permitted the local community members to facilitate other interested groups.

Copies of the educational resource were sent to associated statutory and voluntary groups for their comments. Recommendations led to appropriate modifications. It was acknowledged that research shows that the input of children with respect to accident prevention have often been omitted. Therefore, a series of workshops was developed, including quizzes, group games and competitions, 'spot the danger', and plays, stories and puppet materials, all used to gather information about accidents directly from children.

Community group programme

Initial contact was made with all community groups within the targeted area. Each group was offered a ten-week accident prevention programme. The workshops were carried out within each group's local community and was facilitated by an accident prevention worker, lasted approximately one hour and facilitated between four and fourteen participants at each session. During the 18 months in which the CAPP programme was involved with the community groups, 22 parent groups took part which involved some 542 face-to-face contacts. Each session provided participants with a holistic approach to accidents and their prevention through child development, parental action and environmental components. It also included a first aid session which addressed the groups' concerns about action that might be needed if an accident occurred.

The information and practical interventions followed criteria laid down by the British Red Cross. Evaluation of the workshops was through written comments provided by the group's community manager.

Group development

Following completion of the accident prevention programmes a number of groups identified a need to continue to promote their own personal growth and development. In order to address community needs CAPP employed a twin track strategy including an introduction to components of 'Steps to Excellence' (an approach which developed self-esteem and self-worth); and making contact with an Open Learning Centre which was affiliated to the Advanced Learning System Ltd (providing groups with courses that develop new skills and support the development of self-worth and self-esteem).

Summer safety circus

The development of the summer safety circus was to address the children's needs for accident prevention. As childhood accidents predominantly occur within the home, street and leisure setting and are multifaceted in nature, the intervention required a number of levels. The approach used was within a health promotion ethos and targeted primary school children in relation to three pertinent accidents which had been identified through CAPP research. These accidents included falls, burns and scalds, and road and street accidents.

The summer safety circus was attended by over 300 children and was divided into three distinct units, each relating to a particular accident. The theme centred around two child characters known as Amber and Lance (these characters were developed into puppets and as characters in work booklets for the younger children). Each accident related to specific events in these characters' lives. Throughout the circus the children were actively encouraged to take part in the dramas. Circus performers provided displays at intervals and information was further reinforced by work booklets which were provided. Expertise from members of the inter-agency group was used with information being supplemented by members of the police and the fire brigade who actively took part in performances. Teacher work packs were also provided as a supplement for the teachers who accompanied the pupils.

The road safety campaign

The road safety campaign was carried out in conjunction with a burns and scalds intervention in another school. Questionnaires were developed for use in both inter-ventions. Each area acted as a control group for the other. In a pre-test, the pupils were asked to identify how certain accidents could occur with respect to burns, scalds, fires, and road safety. This information provided baseline data. The initiative was developed in conjunction with the Play in the Environment Group, a multi-agency group comprising private, public and local representatives. The aim of the group was to consult the local community and to put in place traffic calming measures to influence driver behaviour and thereby make urban streets safer. This intervention consisted of members of the CAPP team visiting each of the primary schools and performing a road safety play to the pupils. However, before visiting the school a consultation with a road safety education officer for the Department of the Environment took place to ensure that all information was correct. Teachers and pupils were then supplied with age-related work booklets that pertained to the play. The booklets were developed in consultation with teachers to ensure that they were user-friendly and could be incorporated into the curriculum.

Evaluation

Follow-up analysis using a questionnaire two months after the initial intervention found that 252 pupils had heard a CAPP talk about accidents and the findings produced interesting results. The results illustrated in Figure 4.1 show that in relation to burns and scalds 65 more pupils were able to correctly identify all the named causative objects. There was also an increase in the number of pupils who reported that they would get the fire brigade out and stay out of their home in the case of a fire. There was also an increase in the number of pupils identifying the correct first aid treatment for burns and scalds. When asked who was the safest person to cross the road with, a further 27 pupils identified their parent. The question relating to the safest place to cross had an increase of 55 pupils correctly identifying the zebra crossing and 22 more pupils correctly answering the safest place to play as the pavement. A further 65 pupils stated that they would keep on walking until they reached a zebra crossing.

To ensure that the intervention was not solely seen as a 'school intervention', a poster competition was organized within local community groups. In keeping with the community ethos, the prizes to the winners of this competition brought together the local community, professionals and voluntary bodies.

Immediate successful outcomes

- Within these programmes CAPP has entered into communication with the community providing a forum for the identification of needs in relation to accidents and their prevention.
- The Child Accident Prevention Project provided an awareness of accident prevention in a community setting by building *effective partnerships* involving all the main agencies that have a role to play in preventing accidents. These included a range of agencies such as the police, the schools, the education boards, the

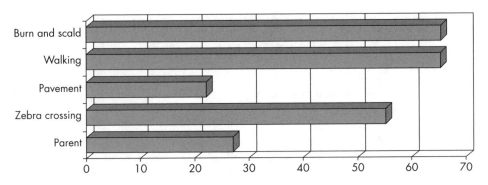

Figure 4.1   Follow-up results two months post initial intervention, Childhood Accident Prevention Programme

housing executive, the fire brigade, local employers, voluntary organisations, media, consultants, nurses, midwives, community nurses, NHS accident and emergency departments, safety officers, environmentalists, and others. This strong inter-agency involvement from key people allowed networking with other agencies and pooling of resources and expertise with respect to accident prevention.

- *Inter-agency working* is often complex and operates at different levels both within and between organizations. The programme highlights a wide range of activities that make up health promotion and need a correspondingly wide range of skills.
- Many organizations can empower their staff and other organizations to work together to serve the community. Also CAPP showed that working together successfully requires the skills to influence others and to develop a shared ownership of programmes and interventions. Most importantly, the intervention convinced potential partners and the local communities that it is worthwhile investing in accident prevention.
- The project has raised awareness of accidents and how they can be prevented in a young population.

Future of the intervention

The Childhood Accident Prevention Programme is an innovative programme developed to address the high incidence of childhood accidents. While the first phase of the project provided knowledge on local accident patterns the second phase used this information to initiate intervention programmes. Whilst the overall objective of increasing awareness of accident risk and stimulation of an increased involvement in accident prevention have been met, it is envisaged that the long-term objective will be to extend the content and scope of the project by building on the experience and skills gained through the intervention. To this end a proposal for further funding has been developed to allow stronger links with the community and the targeting of the elderly population in the area. Healthy alliances and inter-agency working provides a significant contribution to health gain for local populations by making alliances between local agencies, representatives of local people, health service providers, and voluntary and statutory organizations.

Characteristics of best practice in the Childhood Accident Prevention Project

- decisions based on needs assessment
- research-based project
- involving local people and children
- encourage the local residents and community groups to focus and integrate their energies towards goals which decrease the level of accidents in the whole community
- working in partnerships between professionals, agencies and local communities

■ positive community development approach
■ planned approach to working with and training the community
■ empowering and facilitating people, children and the community
■ user-friendly materials for children and schools
■ cross-community working
■ inter-agency networking and disseminating results
■ monitoring, evaluation and report writing
■ bid for further funding.

3 EMPOWERMENT

Preparation for Parenthood Project with Chinese Mothers

Healthcare workers in many communities are aware that social issues such as unemployment, poverty, deprivation, loneliness, culture, bad housing, fear of crime and family disputes have an overriding influence on people's health. Indeed, these can swamp the beneficial effect of improved lifestyle issues such as smoking cessation, diet and exercise. Practitioners within the interventions were clear about using the empowerment model of health promotion which aims to build up the capacity of individuals to make choices, give them control over their own lives and assist them in influencing their environment. Effective health promotion for the nursing professional must require the empowerment of individuals and communities in determining their own destinies and taking on direct involvement in the process of change.

Encouraging local people to become involved in health development means changing their attitude and that of professionals to allow an active participation in efforts to improve their own and others' health. Rathwell (1992) illustrates that in some cases professionals can prevent active participation by the community. In this respect empowerment involves new methods and concepts that can improve the quality and effectiveness of face-to-face health promotion. Several of the projects emphasized the need to involve local people and cultural groups in the decision-making on both setting up an initiative/intervention and fulfilling the aims and objectives of the schemes. Introducing democratic principles into local action is easier in theory than in practice. People in a deprived context not only lack material benefits but also the opportunity to become involved in decisions themselves. This example sees midwives and managers in a hospital antenatal clinic extending their role to assess the cultural needs of the increasing number of Chinese pregnant women in the community and preparing them for a safe labour and parenthood. The intervention was initiated as a 'normative' need based on a professional view. It is also described as a 'felt' need as this minority group of Chinese women feel isolated and lonely in the antenatal setting due to barriers of language and culture.

Targeting health and social need

The midwives in the antenatal clinic suggested that information should be made available for this ethnic minority group in relation to their childbirth needs and expectations. The Midwives Code of Practice (1995) states that: 'Midwives must be able to communicate effectively with women and their families if they are to fulfil their role as documented'.

How the intervention works – the importance of the delivery agent

The assistance of a voluntary interpreter from the Chinese Welfare Association has been invaluable in working with the language and cultural barriers of this ethnic group. The interpreter, and a qualified social worker from Hong Kong, were contacted through Barnardo's and the Chinese Welfare Association. As the interpreter was married and had a family, it was felt that she would be able to relate to these women in pregnancy and labour terms and would also understand the emotional changes that occur. With the aid of the interpreter the midwife was able to communicate effectively with these mothers and develop an understanding of their cultural differences.

Four one-hour sessions are conducted within a relaxed atmosphere to allow the mothers time to grasp and understand the information that is being given to them. The groups are deliberately kept small to encourage trust and openness and the development of a warm and friendly atmosphere. During these sessions the Chinese mothers are usually accompanied by their partners or a friend. As little family support can be given to the mothers in the form of crèche facilities the sessions are organized at a time when other children are at school and when their partners are free to attend. The nature of their employment and hours of working has to be taken into consideration, e.g. being self-employed, employed as cooks and chefs.

Aims and objectives

By using an interpreter the main aims of the teaching sessions are to:

- empower the minority group with information about parentcraft in a way that is culturally appropriate and that they can understand
- identify the group's needs, expectations, fears and anxieties regarding pregnancy and its outcome
- plan a series of short teaching sessions on 'Preparation for Parenthood'
- have information leaflets printed in the Chinese language
- increase Chinese mothers' knowledge of how to keep healthy during pregnancy, labour, the postnatal period and provide information on childcare and infant feeding
- provide health professionals with a better understanding of the minority group's different cultural needs.

The objectives are that:

- by the end of the series of 'Preparation for Parenthood' sessions the Chinese mothers will be empowered and able to make informed choices with regard to their care in the antenatal, labour and postnatal period
- Chinese mothers will have access to relevant issues regarding pregnancy in a language that they can understand
- their understanding of pregnancy and labour will be enhanced
- every Chinese mother will be confident and competent to put the advice into practice
- every Chinese mother will have the opportunity to discuss and question any anxieties or worries with their midwife.

The midwife also looks at some of the terminologies that are used within the context of labour and delivery and rephrases them in a way that this special group of mothers can understand. She has learned a number of Chinese phrases and has developed an interest in Chinese cultural traditions and this has allowed her to understand and respect their customs. In so doing the midwife has broken down barriers of communication. This is particularly important as Chinese mothers are usually reserved and shy people. With the help of the interpreter, the teaching sessions introduce self-explanatory posters on labour, delivery and postnatal health for mother and baby. The sessions consist mainly of discussions and talks about parentcraft. Printed leaflets written in Chinese which cover many topics such as 'Keeping Healthy during Pregnancy' and 'cot death' are given out.

Evaluation

Owing to the language barrier an evaluation questionnaire was not considered suitable. However, the midwife with the help of an interpreter conducts a verbal one-to-one discussion with each participant at the end of the sessions. She also observes the mothers' responses during each teaching session. A follow-up interview with the Chinese mother's named midwife is undertaken to assess how well she has coped in labour and whether she has implemented details from the teaching sessions.

The interviewer asks the named midwife if the mother:

- had a healthy pregnancy
- was able to recognize the signs of labour
- appeared relaxed and in control of her labour
- used relaxation techniques taught by the physiotherapist
- was confident in handling her baby in the postnatal ward
- understands the importance of contraception.

The answers to these questions allow the midwife to adjust the teaching programme to correspond to the needs of the pregnant Chinese woman and further develop the health and social wellbeing of mother and baby.

Immediate successful outcomes

Thanks to the introduction of the intervention midwives in the hospital are now aware of the special needs of the Chinese pregnant woman. For example:

- one main cultural need for a Chinese woman in labour is that she should never be asked to drink water as this is thought to destroy her kidneys and produce a fever. Midwives are now aware of this need and the mother is never asked to drink water. Other cultural needs are that the mother will not take a bath after delivery and will not undress in front of anyone other than her partner.
- the intervention is providing a service and empowering this ethnic minority group, e.g. cot deaths are almost unheard of in Hong Kong because most mothers breastfeed their babies. Within our Western society less women breastfeed and our incidence of cot death is much higher. The intervention shows that it is important that these mothers are made aware of cot death and the measures that they should use to avoid it.
- As these Chinese mothers are not living within an extended family network they are now experiencing more difficulties with breastfeeding and this needs to be supported.

Identified problems

- Serious lack of resources for the publication of teaching material in the Chinese language. There is a need for more information to be printed and available to the mothers.
- Most of the work is being undertaken in the midwife's own free time.
- Limited support from the multidisciplinary team.
- The interpreter should teach the staff more about Chinese cultural background.

The teaching sessions give the midwives and health educators the opportunity to learn about different cultures, including what is acceptable and what is not. The sessions aim to give these Chinese mothers a standard of care that will enable them to feel empowered and less isolated, frightened and distressed. Having a baby is seen as the biggest challenge a couple will ever experience therefore the inclusion of appropriate teaching sessions will make it less frightening and stressful for this minority group and allow the experience for mothers and their partners to be memorable and fulfilling.

Characteristics of best practice in Preparation for Parenthood Project with Chinese Mothers

- decisions based on needs assessment
- planned approach to working with an ethnic minority
- working in partnership with a voluntary agency

- realistic aims
- overcoming resistance and lack of support
- allowing informed choice
- enhancing understanding
- flexible programme meeting the needs of the Chinese families
- providing information and resources in the Chinese language
- breaking down communication and cultural barriers
- empowering women in an ethnic minority and fostering personal growth
- playing an active role in improving the health of Chinese women and their babies in the local community
- strengthening the capacity to cope with labour, delivery and the postpartum
- reducing anxiety and stress in the antenatal period among an ethnic minority
- development of self-esteem
- providing health professionals with a better understanding of the minority group's different cultural needs
- monitoring and evaluation.

4 RESEARCH-BASED

Pre-admission teaching sessions for women before major gynaecological surgery

Research is concerned with generating new knowledge and new approaches that have general application to the health and wellbeing of both individuals and communities. To increase the knowledge base about effectiveness and cost effectiveness and to encourage 'best practice' nurses and healthcare professionals need evidence not only from research but also information about patterns of care, population needs and the availability of resources. It is essential to know what works but also essential to know what is ineffective. This means that practice and service delivery must be based on a firm foundation of research and development with the use of standardized questionnaires and reliable information from evidence-based practice. The following example shows that in a medical world obsessed with technology, nurses and healthcare professionals are being asked to treat the person and not just the disease. Research-based practice is promoted as optimizing the quality of patient care and has shown that if a patient is given adequate information about their surgery, stress is reduced and recovery is enhanced. Dumas (1983) states that: 'the significance of nurses' contribution towards helping man obtain or maintain optimum health lies in his/her ability to facilitate the prevention , mitigation or alleviation of stress'.

Targeting health and social need

Women attending hospital-based pre-operative gynaecological surgery teaching sessions are unique individuals with differing circumstances, backgrounds and cultures. By offering this hospital-based service the staff are offering the 'whole person' care, cognizant of their history, their illness, their coping strategies, their biopsychosocial needs and their dependency and need for support.

Aims and objectives

Following a literature review which confirmed the conviction that lack of knowledge was contributing to increased levels of anxiety for women coming into hospital for gynaecological surgery, nurses working in the ward defined their aims and objectives as a commitment to:

- reducing anxiety and stress in women undergoing major gynaecological surgery
- empowering and optimizing the women's pre-admission health and answer any questions
- speeding recovery and producing good outcomes for patients.

The objectives including the initiation of the teaching programme on a monthly basis; the definition of a standard against which the programme could be audited; and knowledge of the sessions to be communicated to other disciplines and to nursing colleagues, clerical staff, medical and outpatient staff. These aims and objectives followed the process from perceived need (problem), to intervention (pre-admission clinic), to evaluation (standard and audit).

Initiation of the service

The initiation of the pre-admission teaching sessions followed a clearly defined process. Firstly, the process recognized that many women admitted for major surgery were very stressed and often had no idea what to expect, how long they would be in hospital, and whether they would be in much pain. Nurses working in this area identified their needs as a lack of knowledge and advice and a need for support and teaching. Women did not seem to realize that they could be more empowered by taking responsibility towards optimizing their own health. Many were smokers and overweight – factors which could contribute to a delayed recovery. Secondly, the concept of the pre-admission service epitomized both the scientific and human elements of nursing. The scientific component had its basis in research and the human element came from a genuine concern felt by the staff in the gynaecological wards for their patients.

The idea was a collaborative one with commitment from the nursing, medical, physiotherapy and dietician services. Contact was made through the medical records staff as they would be involved in sending out the invitations to patients to attend the teaching sessions, one month before their booked admission. Gynaecology outpatient staff also agreed to inform all patients of the existence of the service and to display posters advertising it. Letters were sent to medical staff, the social worker, the dietician, nurse management, physiotherapy management, the outpatients department and to medical records. An interdisciplinary staff meeting was held to discuss the way forward. This meeting is usually attended by only senior experienced nursing staff and physiotherapists specially trained in gynaecological surgery.

How the intervention works

The programme has been in operation for several years. It has been very successful and uptake has averaged around 70% of women coming into hospital. Nursing staff have reported a marked reduction in anxiety in those patients who attend. Verbal feedback from patients has also been very positive. The pre-admission sessions are now held monthly, usually on a Friday afternoon, 2–4 pm. At each teaching session the physiotherapist talks about anaesthesia and its effects on the respiratory system and stresses the importance of not smoking and how to carry out deep breathing exercises before surgery. Post-operative pain is also discussed and how to cough without causing too much discomfort. She demonstrates lower limb exercises and explains that the importance of early mobility is important for a speedy recovery.

Nursing staff highlight issues such as the process of admission; the patient's expected length of stay in hospital; pain control; strategies for reducing levels of anxiety; the concept of primary nursing care; and the patient's pattern of recovery and rehabilitation.

The dietician talks about healthy eating and emphasizes how a balanced diet can contribute to a speedy recovery and improved wound healing. The women are also taken on a visit to the theatre suites and shown the recovery wards. The session closes with a visit to the wards.

Evaluation

The intervention is being subjected to on-going research and evaluation. One hundred patients were randomly selected and asked to complete an anonymous questionnaire before their discharge from the ward. In the questionnaire the patient is asked if she had attended the pre-operative teaching sessions. If she had then she is asked whether the intervention made her feel less anxious because of her visit. The results are collated, presented regularly and discussed with staff. Initial evaluation has demonstrated a high degree of satisfaction from the patients for the service. The project aims have been achieved and the teaching sessions have had an effect on stress levels. Patients appear to be better prepared for admission; for example, some women have managed to stop smoking or have reduced their smoking habit before surgery. From the questionnaire responses 50% of the women described themselves as 'anxious' and the other half as 'fairly anxious' before surgery. The majority stated that the sessions had helped to reduce their anxiety and the most helpful part had been the knowledge of what was going to happen and meeting the staff. All women felt that it was very helpful to know their primary nurse and felt:

- better prepared both physically and psychologically before surgery
- less anxious
- more empowered
- less likely to experience post-operative complications
- more likely to have a speedier recovery with shorter stay in hospital and better outcomes.

Immediate successful outcomes

- Several patients have managed to stop or reduce their smoking before major surgery. This is reducing the risk of post-operative complications and helping wound healing.
- The ward's innovative intervention is seen as a model for other units.
- The nursing staff in the ward have lifted research out of academic isolation and into the reality of clinical practice.
- Improved practice has resulted in better patient care, enhanced outcomes, empowered patients, increased patient satisfaction and a more rewarding therapeutic relationship between patient and nurse.
- The team have produced a video that outlines all types of information that would be given at the teaching sessions. The video is particularly valuable for women who cannot attend the hospital sessions perhaps because of disability or limited access to transport as it allows these women to gain information and reassurance in their own homes.

These outcomes in themselves make the intervention effective and cost-effective. As a result, there is increased patient and staff satisfaction and the discharge planning process is easier. The clinic is not remaining static as staff are proposing to develop this service to include women who are having laparoscopic investigations and other diagnostic procedures.

Characteristics of best practice in the pre-admission teaching sessions for women before major gynaecological surgery

- motivated, committed and skilled multidisciplinary staff
- practice-based with a firm foundation of research
- decisions based on needs assessment
- empowering women
- realistic aims
- team working with shared goals and objectives
- use of effective and cost-effective methods
- consumer involvement
- playing an active role in improving the post-operative health of women
- reducing anxiety and stress among women patients
- allowing women to take increasing control which is central to good health promotion
- disseminating results
- evaluation, monitoring and audit.

5 MULTIDISCIPLINARY WORKING

Healthcare project for single homeless people

Reducing inequalities in health must be a team activity in which nurses work with many other disciplines and professions. No single profession has a monopoly on health promotion or is equipped to perform all the necessary tasks. Many of the case studies illustrate the 'best practice' of working within a multidisciplinary context. Primary healthcare nursing involves the use of extensive teamwork and multidisciplinary activities. Nurses and midwives within the hospital setting might contribute by being involved in activities over and above their bedside health education interaction with patients.

There is a need to undertake new ways of working which are consistent with health promotion concepts and principles. These involve the creation of supportive health environments and promote collaborative working in multidisciplinary teams with specialist input from social workers, psychologists, doctors, physiotherapists and dieticians etc. Such groups have both a supportive and educative function and nurses provide roles as initiators, facilitators and contributors. One case study, cited above, illustrates the establishment of groups at pre-admission giving nurses and other professionals the insight into the experiences that patients are likely to encounter during their admission and patients' knowledge requirements for the rehabilitation process. Another intervention shows midwives and physiotherapists working together with groups of Chinese mothers and assisting them through an interpreter to identify their needs in pregnancy, labour and delivery. The following example illustrates district nursing teams, social workers and GPs all working to improve the health and social wellbeing of the homeless.

Targeting health and need

District nursing teams have recognized a growing need for single homeless men and women to receive health education and information about the range of primary healthcare services available to them. After discussion with nursing management and social services, a district nursing team from an inner city health clinic commenced a health promotion programme to empower homeless people. This took the form of a monthly visit to individual residents of Green House, a lodging accommodation for homeless men, to deal with health issues such as GP registration, blood pressure, feet care, chiropody, eye testing, dental care, weight, cholesterol, medication dosage and safe and proper disposal of out of use medicine. The assessment also included correct referrals to community specialists and professions allied to medicine as appropriate.

A similar programme was then introduced into a community hostel within the city. It became apparent that the needs of this group were more acute as it included young male and female homeless people awaiting resettlement. At this point the district nursing team felt that it was necessary to address and meet the social, emotional and economic needs concerning the homeless and their carers by creating a Single Homeless Healthcare Project. The project was funded by a voluntary organization and developed with the establishment of an advisory group composed of multidisciplinary professionals whose remit was to consider specific issues and provide a working knowledge of existing policies towards the homeless.

Aims and objectives

The aims and objectives of the Single Homeless Healthcare Project are to:

- improve the health status of single homeless people living in target hostel accommodation
- facilitate and promote single homeless people's access to local mainstream healthcare services
- provide health screening to establish basic health status
- provide district nursing care to hostel residents when the need arises and the opportunity is there
- empower single homeless people to make informed choices about their health needs
- offer a training programme to hostel workers on health issues
- develop a health education programme that is client led and specifically geared to meet their needs
- increase the healthcare skills and knowledge of the multidisciplinary team
- conduct a research survey which will look at the general health status of single homeless people and the statutory and voluntary services they use
- evaluate the project.

How the intervention works

The project now assesses the healthcare needs of residents in four major hostels for the homeless in the city. The programme consists of one-to-one health screening offering basic information on health problems and health education sessions that cover a range of topics. Input to these sessions is from both the statutory services and the voluntary sector. To remove cultural barriers and facilitate and promote single homeless people's access to local mainstream services, the programme encourages and assists hostel residents to register with a local doctor and make use of their services, and to access other health services. It also encourages doctors and dentists to accept homeless people. Help from relevant healthcare professionals is facilitated by bringing the service to the resident, e.g. the client with learning disabilities.

The project calculates the number and percentage of residents who have registered with local doctors and dentists; and attended doctors and dentists in the previous six months. The district nursing team are empowering single homeless people to make informed choices about their health needs by making regular screening available in hostels, and by providing information to residents on ways to improve their health. The team provides health education related to lifestyle issues to residents, e.g. alcohol, drugs, sex education. The team monitors uptake by calculating the number and percentage of:

- residents who have been screened
- specific health improvements at follow-up clinics or screening

- self assessment of health improvements and awareness of option.

The nursing and social work team are also increasing the healthcare skills and knowledge of support staff including carers by providing training for groups of hostel staff, together with general health education and health promotion where possible. The team identify the number of health-related training sessions delivered/facilitated and the number of staff volunteers attending health sessions. Training given to participants is evaluated by the team. The team also records the number of staff/volunteers gaining healthcare-related accreditation e.g. in first aid, food hygiene/safety, AIDS awareness, drugs/alcohol/solvents, women's issues.

Evaluation

The health education sessions are evaluated at the end of each session using an evaluation questionnaire form. The numbers of clients who receive health screening and the increase in GP registration are counted monthly. Evaluation of the programme highlighted a number of performance targets that the project considered for the year 1996–1997. During this period the project has:

- Increased the level of registration (including temporary registration) with local GP practices by 10%.
- Screened 40% of all residents in the hostels during the period from October 1996 to March 1997.
- Provided for the individual healthcare needs of 50% of hostel residents.
- Developed and implemented a general package of training on healthcare needs of single homeless people, aimed at residents and staff of all agencies.

Intermediate successful outcomes

- The provision of health education has enabled a number of single homeless people to become empowered and make informed choices about their health and access to services.
- Hostel workers are provided with advice and support on health issues, through the provision of a nursing contact person.
- An increase in GP registration of single homeless people has been achieved.
- An improved communication structure between the statutory and voluntary services involved in homeless issues has been created.

Identified problems

- Cultural barriers still exist as many GPs and dentists are cautious about registering a homeless person with their practice.
- There are difficulties in following-up treatments due to the transient nature of the client group.

Future of the intervention

There are a number of potential areas for future development of the project. The inter-agency working and multidisciplinary collaboration of the project will provide an opportunity to increase understanding of the broader cultural needs and issues that are affecting homeless people. The relevance of larger multidisciplinary teams to cover homeless areas has been indicated.

The health education element of the programme could be incorporated into a homeless resettlement programme, and the development of client-held records would provide continuity and ease of access to health information. The project itself will provide invaluable learning resources for multi-professional undergraduate and postgraduate nursing and social science students.

Characteristics of best practice in a healthcare project for single and homeless people

- decisions based on needs assessment
- planned non-judgmental approach to working with the homeless
- health alliances and inter-agency networking
- empowering homeless people to make informed choices about their health and social needs
- team-working with shared goals and objectives
- offering a training programme to hostel workers on health issues
- increasing knowledge, healthcare skills to both the homeless and their carers
- playing an active role in improving the health of homeless people in the local community
- introducing a referral system to community specialists and PAMS as appropriate
- strengthening the capacity of homeless people to cope with health-related problems
- reducing anxiety and stress among homeless people and their carers
- offering support to the homeless
- providing access to a GP and health services
- monitoring and evaluation.

6 NEEDS ASSESSMENT

Assessment of health and social needs in the older person

A number of the examples examined the involvement of the community and individuals in the process of identifying needs and identifying gaps in evidence-based practice and service delivery. There was evidence of successful work on community needs health profiling to inform a population view of health needs. Others were responding to a perceived need for a more flexible provision and were offering a change of location, time or availability of the service. In response to a general need for a wider range of information concerning health issues, all the interventions engaged in different forms of dissemination, ranging from conferences, roadshows, workshops, seminars, to circuses, fairs, user-friendly literature for a minority group, advice centres, telephone helplines, drop-in centres, counselling, lay health workers, and information videos.

Community action is when members of communities work together to demand changes in their environment or in the services delivered in order to improve their health. Local government agencies are working in collaboration with local communities on the shared agenda of enabling improvements to the wellbeing and quality of life of local people by needs assessment. The following is an example of a project that was initiated to develop a partnership with a local community organization and to identify certain needs and respond sensitively in meeting them.

Targeting health and need

The Bridgecare project is a three-year partnership between statutory and voluntary agencies which is developing locally based individually tailored services for older people. It is sensitive to local needs, provides employment within the community, and improves the quality of life for the elderly population within the area. It is part of a network of services and activity schemes provided by its parent organization. Through anecdotal evidence and feedback through the area's advice centre there appeared to be a need for a more consistent and comprehensive programme for the older people within this inner city area.

Aims and objectives

The aims and objectives of the project were to:

- develop a pilot programme of service provision to meet needs identified through a health and social care assessment
- develop a methodology for assessing the health and social care needs of the older person within the community
- examine the patterns of health and social care needs and develop methods for prioritizing and translating these into appropriate responses
- develop a pilot programme of service provision to meet needs identified through the health and social care assessment.

Bridgecare views these aims and objectives within a holistic view of older person care, one which addresses the mental as well as the physical and understands that an assortment of variables can impinge upon an older person's health and social wellbeing as well as their quality of life. This eclectic approach to healthcare recognizes the centrality of imaginative and innovative health promotion as part of an integrated programme rather than an adjunct to it. The ethos acknowledges the importance of social interaction in forging new social networks and strengthening established ones, as well as reducing isolation and the incidence of depression.

The assessment of health and social needs in the older person

The aims of the first phase of the project were to identify the need for health and social care for those over 75-years old in the area. To identify their particular needs, a methodology had to be identified and tested in the area. A further aim was to evaluate the effectiveness of individual goal setting and attainment in the care of the older person and to test its use in assessing population need. Finally, methods for translating information on needs into appropriate responses had to be developed.

A research nurse needs assessor was appointed to develop appropriate methodologies for assessing the social and health needs of the older person population in the area so that service provision could be tailored to identified need. The European Prototype for Integrated Care (EPIC) Assessment (EASY Questionnaire) was developed as the main instrument of needs assessment. A few additional questions were added to include details of living arrangements, formal services, financial support, depression and morale. It is a tool that could successfully be used by a variety of agencies and professionals and act as a model for future needs assessments in other targeted areas. As a screening instrument it allowed the development of a comprehensive assessment of need for the target group.

Part 1 of the project is a survey of the health and social needs of the elderly population and the Department of Health Care for the Older Person at the University of Sheffield has been commissioned to analyse the results.

Part 2 of the project highlights the unmet need identified by the elderly people themselves during the study.

Target group

There are approximately 600 over-75s in the area and the sample of 187 individuals interviewed was identified from GP's over-75 assessment lists. The researcher (a qualified nurse) interviewed the sample as part of their annual health check. All interviews were conducted in the person's home and sometimes in the presence of the carer. For those in residential accommodation a room was used to allow privacy.

The sample of 187 older people were randomly allocated to two groups. The first group were asked to complete Section E of the EASY Questionnaire (Needs, Goals, Outcomes). To introduce this section and identify the individual's wish or 'need', the following question was used: 'If there was one thing which may be done to improve things for you and make your life easier or better, what would it be?'

The second group of interviewees completed Section E of EASY at the six-month follow-up visit. A natural sub-division of the groups occurred and these have been followed through to the conclusion of the study.

Results

A total of 98 older people were asked about unmet need in the first round of visits. In their responses 54.08% said that they had no unmet needs, whereas 45.92% identified a need, or in some cases, several needs. For many of the participants their needs required the provision of a specialist service, equipment or the involvement of several agencies. In total 60 patients with identified needs required 74 referrals. A breakdown of total needs and referrals are illustrated in Figures 4.2 and 4.3.

The study shows that in assessing the older person it is important to ask the right questions. An extensive health check can be undertaken but few of the client's true

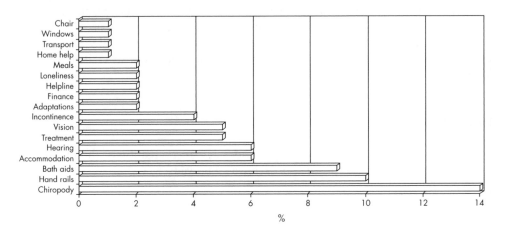

Figure 4.2 Summary of needs identified in Woodstock Ward

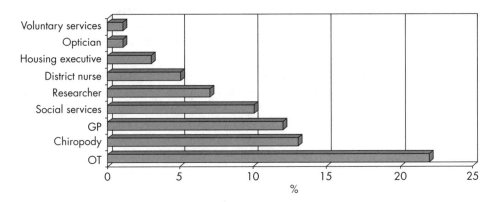

Figure 4.3 Summary of referrals made in Woodstock Ward

needs identified. All the participants in this study received a health assessment as previously described but the amount of unmet need was much greater in the group directly asked about their needs.

The six-inch hearing test that is part of the assessment is said to be a sensitive test of significant hearing impairment in the older person. However, it is interesting to note that self-reported hearing difficulty (in the context of a lot of people talking together) was more common than failure to pass the hearing test. This discrepancy suggests that mild forms of hearing impairment are a major problem for the older person. Practitioners working with older people should be aware of the need to talk clearly and directly and try to reduce background noise. Moreover, loneliness and depression are often associated with hearing loss in older people. Figure 4.2 shows that psychological difficulties were common among this sample group with 30% reporting some degree of loneliness and 26% having elevated scores in the clinical depression range of the Geriatric Depression Scale. On the other hand, many others were reporting high levels of morale indicating a wide range of psychological wellbeing among this population.

Cognitive impairment in severe form only affected 1% of the population and behavioural problems and problems with carers were low. About two-thirds of the population were living on their own and of these one-third received visits from family and friends only once a week or less. The research suggests that social visiting might prove beneficial given the confirmation of relatively high levels of social isolation and loneliness.

Evaluation

An external agency was commissioned to undertake an evaluation of the Bridgecare project and a proposed five-phase approach was followed:

- Scoping exercise
- Evaluation of needs assessment
- Linking needs assessment with service delivery
- Impact of responses to needs assessment
- Global evaluation.

The evaluation process was flexible and sensitive to the requirements of the project's development. The evaluator's conclusions are that the needs assessment phase of the project provides both the foundation and structure from which the project as a whole can develop and evolve. The use of the structured approach to needs assessment, based on the EPIC Assessment System, has proven useful in establishing the project among respondents as well as in the general area. The success in creating a positive climate for the project should encourage, and permit, the use of less structured approaches within the overall needs assessment process.

Immediate successful outcomes

- The project belongs to the community and is of the community
- The committee is democratic, two of its members representing the target population in the area

- The project is a voluntary, non-profit making organization, which means that quality rather than cost determine both decision-making and policy
- It is committed to a holistic approach to health and social need which recognizes the need for flexibility of both activities and timetabling
- It raised an awareness of health and social issues for example, the very high rate of depression in the area (26.2% of the total sample). It also identified the long waiting list for occupational therapy (previously 8 months; the target now in place is for a 3-month maximum waiting time).
- Various agencies have made an impact in this project. Housing Executive has been given information collated on housing and housing needs. The Benefits Agency has been informed of the problems getting information on benefits. The Department of the Environment (Transport Section) information has been given on transport in general and public transport in particular. The Royal Mail are awaiting planning permission to site a new posting facility within the area due to the high density of older people.

Individual outcomes

Outcomes in this section were identified by the older people, at their six-month follow-up visit:

- Two people who had been unable to use their telephones for several years are now in regular contact with their families, and no longer need someone to answer their telephone for them. This was achieved because the research nurse asked BT to change their telephones.
- Four people received help with claim forms for benefits, permitting purchase of appropriate support, preserving self-esteem.
- Twenty-two people received occupational therapy interventions which increased safety and independence levels for them.
- Thirteen people received chiropody intervention to keep their feet pain- and infection-free, promoting mobility and independence.
- Twelve people were referred to their GPs, some for cataract operations to restore their eyesight, some due to confusion about their medication which, when sorted promoted their psychological wellbeing.
- Ten people were referred to social services for a day centre placement, home help, telephone helpline or advice. Outcomes were reduced loneliness, adequate nutrition, increased safety, increased knowledge and improved psychological wellbeing.

Characteristics of best practice in the assessment of health and social needs of the older person

- decisions based on needs assessment
- identifying unmet needs
- research-based project
- model for future needs assessment
- involving local older people
- service provision sensitive to local needs
- viewing partnership with community agencies as a shared resource seeking to improve the social and health status of clients
- providing employment in the community
- providing a quality homecare service
- reducing inequalities in health and social care of the older person
- playing an active role in improving the health and quality of life of the elderly population
- empowerment
- reducing anxiety and depression
- reducing levels of loneliness and offering support networks
- reducing waiting list for occupational therapy
- developing an innovative research methodology for assessing the health and social needs within the community
- strengthening the capacity to cope
- use of cost-effective methods
- disseminating results and information sharing
- monitoring and evaluation.

7 COMMUNITY DEVELOPMENT

A community Home from Hospital Service

Several interventions used community development as a commitment to a holistic approach to health and social need that recognizes the central importance of social inclusion, social support and social networks. Individuals and communities need to be fully involved in partnerships and networks to set priorities, make decisions, plan strategies and implement them in order to achieve better health. Many interventions used the community action model which aims to mobilize disadvantaged communities to reduce the fact that inequalities may damage their health. An indicator of 'best practice' is illustrated by those nurses, midwives and health visitors who enable people to make choices about healthier lifestyles, as well as facilitate greater access to screening and treatment services. In similar holistic vein, health promotion agents are offering a wide range of services both directly helping individuals in the community as well as encouraging others to act as lay health promoters. The example shows a voluntary agency called Bryson House that has a lengthy history of pioneering new services in response to emerging need in close collaboration with the statutory sector and the local community. It is within this framework that the 'Home from Hospital Service' is offered.

Targeting Health and Need

The services provided by Bryson House are of a 'family-type' caring nature and as such do not have a remit to provide professional nursing care. The scheme is open to everyone, irrespective of social class, gender, political or religious status and is also supporting vulnerable people by helping them adapt to their own communities and allowing a link to other support structures. Recent government policy changes have had a significant impact on the development of domiciliary services for vulnerable, frail and elderly people.

The Home from Hospital Service provides a bridge between hospital and home as it gives short-term support to people who are adapting to living in the community after a stay in hospital. It was developed as a response to the needs of older people but now accepts referrals for adults, who meet the criteria for referral, on their discharge from hospital. The structure, ethos and training programme of all schemes are the same, but location, size and other aspects of individual schemes may differ according to local needs and resources. Each local scheme is monitored by its own advisory committee consisting of representatives of those responsible for local caring services in hospital and community. In this way the family-type support offered is realistically based and becomes a supplement to appropriate multidisciplinary support. However, in many situations the practical care and emotional support provided by the Home from Hospital care workers for a few weeks may be the only additional support required before the client becomes fully independent. It illustrates new patterns of partnership between statutory and voluntary services that combine and focus knowledge and skills to the benefit of client and services. It has an established induction training programme for all staff with training packages linked to further staff development opportunities and quality assurance procedures.

Aims and objectives

The aims of the services are:

- to assist individuals to make the transition from hospital to home successfully
- to enable patients to return home as soon as possible once their treatment is completed
- to provide intensive practical and emotional support for up to six weeks after discharge
- to enable patients and clients to regain their confidence and to adjust to being at home again and to retain their quality of life
- to provide an additional link between hospital and community services in helping the patient make the transition from hospital to home

- to support and encourage the involvement of informal resources, e.g. relatives, neighbours and friends
- to help prevent unnecessary re-admission to hospital or admission to residential accommodation in the early period of discharge
- to ensure that all necessary community resources are ready before withdrawal of the service.

How the intervention works

The co-ordinator of the relevant Home from Hospital Service visits the patient/client in hospital and explains the service, establishes where there may be anxieties or problems in the early stage following discharge, and introduces the care worker to the patients.

Care workers are then employed to befriend and give family-type support to those adults who are ready for discharge from hospital who either live alone or with a frail relative, and do not have sufficient family or community support. The care workers provide practical help, personal care and emotional support enabling people who are vulnerable to adapt to being at home again. They receive pre-service induction training and on-going in-service training. The care worker normally brings the patient home from hospital, ensuring that there is someone who can settle the patient/client in their home and ease any anxieties. S/he will also check that there is food in the house and that the house is warm.

The time limited nature of the scheme (maximum 6 weeks – usually 2 to 3 weeks) establishes targets for the client, the scheme and the statutory services in terms of achievable physical and social rehabilitation. This has been found to be a valuable tool in assessing the intermediate and likely longer-term service needs of each client more accurately than is normally possible in hospital or immediately on discharge.

Multidisciplinary team work

The contribution to the monitoring and development of schemes from the participating disciplines is invaluable. All are actively involved with service delivery and with their help the client receives not only a more effective service but also inter-agency difficulties can be unravelled and the quality of services enhanced. The Home from Hospital Service, because of its intensive flexibility and support in the early days, has enabled many patients to be resettled at home with formal and informal support systems. Others less able or fortunate have been more ready to accept alternative forms of care having had the opportunity to try being at home with the protection of the scheme. This facility offers a trial period at home illustrating the point that assessment and accurate targeting of scarce resources are valuable aspects of the Home from Hospital Service, as is the enhanced opportunity for client choice.

Intermediate successful outcomes

The programme has undergone a lengthy evaluation and a number of successes have been identified namely:

- the wide community involvement developed through the scheme by providing a bridge from hospital to community
- the provision of a service which gives greater choice and flexibility for dependent individuals
- a partnership agreement with multidisciplinary working which allows the scheme to draw on the professional 'expertise' of both parties
- providing a continuity of care which allows the first contact in hospital (building up trust and confidence) and transfer into the community
- accurate targeting of scarce resources.

Characteristics of best practice in the Home from Hospital Service

- decisions based on needs assessment
- reducing inequalities in health and social care in the elderly and frail
- identifying unmet needs
- bridging a gap in service
- involving local elderly people
- providing choice and flexibility
- service provision sensitive to convalescent needs
- viewing partnership with statutory and voluntary sector
- providing a cost-effective service
- providing a quality homecare service
- playing an active role in improving the quality of life of people returning home from hospital
- empowering individuals and carers
- reducing anxiety and depression after a stay in hospital
- reducing levels of loneliness and offering a support service
- strengthening the capacity of people to cope
- monitoring and evaluation.

---

8   AUDIT AND EVALUATION

A Well Person Clinic for People with Learning Disabilities

Audit is best viewed as a systematic method for improving quality and/or ensuring that healthcare meets the needs of local people. Audit is concerned with judging whether an intervention is working effectively in practice and in further assessing whether or not resources are being used to the best advantage. Findings of an audit relate to the work of a multidisciplinary team, organization, alliance, or programme. Nurses have a clear understanding of the benefits of auditing their practice. Clinical audit is successfully illustrated in several of the case studies, where its presence raised nurses' awareness of their standard of performance and thus effected an improvement in the quality and outcome of patient care. The respondents state that clinical audit provides a framework within which clinical guidelines, needs assessment, evidence of effectiveness and information on cost-effectiveness can all be brought together to improve the quality of patient/client care.

Evaluation can combine the use of qualitative and quantitative methods and examples of these techniques are presented throughout many of the interventions studied. The formative style of evaluation allows ways in which interventions can be improved by concentrating on their process. There is an apparent tendency for evaluators to report only the positive aspects of any project, but the nursing examples of the evaluation process also demonstrate problem areas and therefore give an insight into ways in which the effectiveness of the intervention could be improved. The key to making health and social need interventions more successful is discovering which activities are effective and how to make them even more so. Evaluation is also an important aid to quality assurance and quality of practice. This example clearly illustrates evaluation in practice.

Targeting health and social need

Health centres have already established Well Person Clinics, where patients are being encouraged to take responsibility for maintaining their good health by presenting themselves for screening. The idea of a more localized service for people with learning disability was based upon the observation that 'few people with learning difficulties wore glasses'. Can we presume that people with learning disabilities all have excellent eyesight or have there been difficulties in taking the person for an eye test? In considering these principles in relation to people with learning disabilities, the Community Nursing Team for Learning Disabilities in the area considered the following:

- People with learning disabilities are entitled to the same range and quality of services as are available to other citizens and to services designed to meet their special needs.
- People with learning disabilities should also have access to health promotion, health education, and programmes of health surveillance.
- Services should adapt to meet the needs of each individual.

Based on this thinking, the community nursing team decided to explore further the establishment of a Well Person Clinic for People with Learning Disabilities. Multi-professional support from colleagues within services for people with learning disability and primary healthcare have been essential in their involvement to sustain this quality project and its future developments. After a consultative process in which the idea was discussed with the programme manager, GP representatives, nursing staff, and the consultant for mental handicap, a questionnaire was designed and sent to a number of carers to give them the opportunity to comment. The overall response from both professionals and carers was very positive towards the idea of a clinic.

How the intervention works

A small pilot study was undertaken with 18 people with learning disabilities. All were screened, all had unidentified and treatable conditions, and several had more than one. The pilot study findings highlighted the difficulties faced by people with learning difficulties in gaining access to mainstream health-screening services:

- Fear of unknown places and investigations, leading to non-cooperation
- Challenging behaviour, such as hyperactivity, shouting or self-injurious behaviour
- Difficulties meeting certain social expectations, such as waiting in queues, behaving appropriately in reception areas and interacting with staff
- Difficulties of professionals in assessing needs owing to insufficient training
- Inability to communicate needs such as pain, discomfort, deficiencies in vision
- Difficulty in reading and understanding published material or technical terms
- Lack of specialist health screening for people with learning disabilities
- Failure of carers or people with learning difficulties to recognize the need for health screening and reluctance to seek medical or nursing attention
- Assumption that changes in behaviour or health are both due to learning disabilities.

These prompted members of the community nursing service to consult with the multi-professional team of carers, local GPs, dentists, chiropodists and opticians to establish a tailored health-screening programme for people with specialized needs. The clinic was established and is held in the local Adult Training Centre as it was felt that the clients would feel more at ease in familiar surroundings. Consent was obtained by using questionnaires which were completed either by the clients themselves or by their carers. Information on particular health concerns was also sought. Before the clinic began each client was asked if they wished to attend. When it was unclear whether the person understood the questions, two nurses demonstrated the relevant procedure.

Aims and objectives

The aims of the project were:

- To provide a first point of entry to health screening which is more accessible to people with learning disabilities and their carers
- To facilitate onward referral to appropriate professionals
- To raise awareness of the health needs of this client group
- To highlight and intervene with treatable health conditions.

Evaluation after two years

Screening clinics are an essential first step in developing a broader-based health promotion strategy for people with learning disabilities. This project has taken three and a half years and has screened 191 people aged between 19 and 65. In total, 176 had previously undetected and treatable conditions, and of those who were identified as being in need of screening most (83%) had more than one condition; only four refused. The nurses conducted the screening in a sensitive manner, taking time to build up a rapport with the client. The procedures carried out varied according to the individual need. Service users had blood pressure, weight and body mass recorded; urine tests on site; urine and blood samples (full blood count, thyroid function and serum cholesterol) taken for analysis; anti-convulsant and lithium levels tested as appropriate; and assessment of hair, eyes and vision, skin, mouth, ears and hearing, breasts and testicles.

If a potential or actual abnormality was discovered an appointment was made with the appropriate member of the primary healthcare team.

Findings of health screening evaluation of 191 people with learning disability

Screening measures	Number and examples of detected conditions
Blood pressure	Hypertension (10), hypotension (13)
Weight	Obese (89), underweight (9)
Mouth	Poor oral hygiene (17), loose teeth (20), irregular formation (4), tooth decay (31), gum infection (6)
Hair	Dandruff (19), dry scalp (11)
Urinalysis	Glucose (1), protein (6), blood (5)
Skin	Dryness (11), varicose veins (6), eczema (2), psoriasis (2), acne (17)
Testicles	Undescended (5), swollen testicles (1), underdeveloped testicles (1)
Feet	Corns (10), hard skin (31), verruca (4), athletes foot, damaged nails (20), poor circulation (3)
Breasts	Inverted nipples (2), tags (1), breast lumps (2), male breast enlargement (2)
Ears	Excess wax (81), hearing difficulties (3)
Eyes	Cataracts (1), reduced vision (35)
Blood tests	Hypothyroidism

The evaluation highlighted differences in health status that varied according to age; the mean number of conditions detected for people aged 19–35 was 2.8, while for people aged over 35 years the mean figure was 3.3 conditions. According to their actual or potential seriousness the conditions were assigned to two categories. For over half (n=277) the conditions (including abnormalities in blood pressure, weight, urine, breasts, testes, ears, eyes and blood results) required medical attention. All the conditions in this category could have been detected in routine GP screening initiatives and would generally be seen as being preventable with appropriate health education. However, they would have remained undetected without screening sessions by the project. Of the problems highlighted some form of intervention or treatment was required from the multi-professional team, either the GP/consultant, nurses, the chiropodist, or the optician.

Many healthcare professionals appear to adopt a complacent approach towards people with learning disabilities. Problems can be seen as trivial compared with the range of difficulties facing this client group and therefore no action is taken. A major obstacle in identifying problems associated with people's breasts or testicles is the assumption that people with learning disabilities are asexual or sexually inactive. Indeed, both of these assumptions may lead to cancers being overlooked. In addition, impaired vision or hearing can hamper a person's ability to perform self-care tasks and may be interpreted as lack of cooperativeness. Abnormalities in a person's skin, mouth, hair and feet should not be minimalized as they may have a major impact on the quality of that person's life. Community nurses working with this client group must work with primary healthcare team colleagues in ensuring these services are available.

Some suggestions for the initial steps in developing a health promotion service for people with special needs include:

- Education to increase awareness among primary healthcare team members
- Increased use of health education with suitable equipment and individually prepared information which suits the sensory and motor abilities of the client group
- Development of health promotion services in all localities which are accessible to people with learning disabilities and are staffed by specialist staff
- At least yearly follow-up for all people with learning disabilities to monitor progress of conditions detected and repeat health screening
- Education for people with learning disabilities and their carers in relation to the need for health promotion, the process of screening and the tests involved
- Ensure adequate services for those aged below 19 years in an attempt to reduce preventable health problems arising in adult life.

Intermediate successful outcomes

The evaluation highlights many benefits to both the client and their carers and to the providers of service with screening, namely:

- The health screening programme is the first of its kind and continues to provide relevant research and evaluation information in assisting the development of services in the UK
- With screening there is less risk of unidentified but treatable conditions/illnesses developing into long-term chronic illnesses. Early detection allows clients to lead a fuller and healthier life
- The service is cost-effective for the provider manager, with long-term financial benefits
- Parent or carer's burden of care is lessened with healthier more able people
- The initiative has become a Quality Standard in the Purchaser Specification for Services for all Health and Social Service Providers
- Working in partnership with various multi-professional groups.

Future of the intervention

A proposal has been developed to pilot the development of a co-ordinated health screening (surveillance) service that will lead to improved healthcare, health promotion and overall health gain for people with a learning disability. If successful this new development will forge links with primary healthcare (GPs) and disability services to improve communication and plan constructive improvements in the holistic care of people with a learning disability.

Characteristics of best practice in the health screening of people with learning disabilities

- motivated committed and skilled multidisciplinary staff
- practice based on a firm foundation of research
- decisions based on needs assessment
- planned approach
- working in partnerships and health alliances
- empowering people with learning disabilities and their carers
- community nursing team working with shared goals and objectives
- use of effective and cost-effective methods
- consumer involvement
- playing an active role in improving the health of people with special needs
- allowing people with learning disabilities to take increasing control which is central to good health promotion
- disseminating results
- monitoring survey methods and audit.

FURTHER READING

Dumas, R.G. (1983) Social, economic and political factors and mental illness. *Journal of Psychosocial Nursing and Mental Health Services*, 21(3): 31–35.

Lazenbatt, A. (1997) *Targeting Health and Social Need, Volume 1: The Contribution of Nurses, Midwives and Health Visitors*. Belfast: The Stationery Office.

Lazenbatt, A. (1999) *Manual for Evaluation and Effectiveness in Practice, Volume 2*. Belfast: The Stationery Office.

Lazenbatt, A. (2000) Tackling inequalities in health in Northern Ireland. *Community Practitioner*, 73(2): 481–483.

Lazenbatt, A. and Hunter, P. (2000) 'An evaluation of a drop-in centre for working women'. Queen's University of Belfast/Royal College of Nursing, Northern Ireland.

Lazenbatt, A. and Orr, J. (2001) Evaluation and effectiveness in practice. *International Journal of Nursing Practice* 7(6) (in press).

Lazenbatt, A., McWhirter, L., Bradley, M. and Orr, J. (1999) The role of nursing partnership interventions in improving the health of disadvantaged women. *Journal of Advanced Nursing*, 30(6): 1280–1288.

Lazenbatt, A., McWhirter, L., Bradley, M. and Orr, J. (2000a) Community nursing achievements in targeting health and social need. *Nursing Times Research* 5(3), 178–192.

Lazenbatt, A., McWhirter, L., Bradley, M., Orr, J. and Chambers, M. (2000b) Tackling inequalities in health and social wellbeing – evidence of 'good practice' by nurses, midwives and health visitors. *International Journal of Nursing Practice*, 6(2) April: 76–88.

Lazenbatt, A., Sinclair, M., Salmon, S. and Calvert, J. (2001a) Telemedicine as a support system to encourage breastfeeding in Northern Ireland: a case study design. *Journal of Telemedicine and Telecare* (in press).

Lazenbatt, A., Lynch, U. and O'Neill, E. (2001b) Revealing the hidden 'troubles' in Northern Ireland: the role of Participatory Rapid Appraisal. *Health Education Research* (in press).

PART TWO

████████████

CHAPTER 5

AN INTRODUCTION TO EVALUATION

WHAT IS EVALUATION?

Remember from the outset that evaluation can be simple and is something that we all do all the time without thinking. We are always judging the importance and value of things. However, many of us make quick judgments and realize that we should be more careful to get the right information and to use it in the right way in order to reach our final judgment. When this happens it makes evaluation more complex. Systematic evaluations are different from everyday evaluation in that they make careful definitions of what is to be evaluated, and of the information needed, as well as careful selection and use of methods for collecting and analysing the information. The literature on evaluation highlights a range of approaches as well as the differences in the questions emphasized by each approach. The evaluator has to know about a range of methods and approaches in order to choose the best method for the purpose of the particular evaluation. To understand any evaluation it is necessary to appreciate some basic terms as listed below.

Evaluator	the person making the evaluation.
Funders/sponsors	those who initiate or pay for the evaluation.
Users	those who are involved in an intervention or who make use of or act on the evaluation.
Intervention	an action on, or an attempt to change, a person, group, community, population or organization which is the subject of the evaluation.
Target	the individual, population or organization which the intervention aims to affect.
Outcome	a broad concept which encompasses a variety of the consequences or that which comes out of the evaluation (outputs) and which can be described as immediate effects, intermediate effects or longer-term outcomes. (We will discuss these differences in Chapter 9, Stages 7–9.)

Many evaluations measure some aspect of a patient, client, community or population before and after an intervention. However, it is important to realize that a number of things apart from the intervention may account for the before–after difference which an evaluation detects. It is therefore important that we look at target outcomes which may correspond more directly to the difference produced and may be attributed to the intervention. Remember that an outcome is the end result of an intervention and is a broad concept which encompasses a variety of consequences, some of which are intended and some are not.

Using the definition of outcome given above we understand that we can only make a value judgment if we make a comparison. In any evaluation these comparisons may include:

- comparing the state (holistic health) of one or more people, groups, organizations or populations
- comparing the needs of people or populations both before and after the intervention
- comparing the objectives of the intervention to the actual achievements
- comparing what is done to a set of standards or guidelines (e.g. audit).

It is also important to understand who makes an evaluation and to assess whether it is an internal or external evaluation. External evaluators are researchers or consultancy units not directly managed by and independent of the sponsor and user of the evaluation. Internal evaluators are evaluation or development units or researchers that are internal to the organization, and that evaluate interventions or services carried out by the organization. Self-evaluation is where practitioners or teams evaluate their own practice so as to improve it.

WHAT CAN YOU EVALUATE?

It is necessary now for most people working for the promotion of health to be able to use, understand, and undertake evaluations. In the health field there are four structured areas that can be evaluated, namely treatments; services and programmes; health and related policies; and changes to health organizations.

Treatments, services, programmes and policies are all 'interventions' which are used to intervene in people's lives in order to improve their health and social well-being. Throughout this handbook we will use the term 'intervention' to denote the above terms. However, they are all different in nature and also have different target groups, e.g.

Treatments may involve a part or whole of a person and include different therapies such as drugs, surgical, physical, psychological, educational and social therapies.
Services may involve communities, target groups or populations and are larger in scope and more complex than treatments. They may include training, education, support, self-help and information-giving processes.
Health policies may involve larger populations and communities and aim to change or regulate how people think and behave. The fact that a policy is being evaluated will influence how managers and practitioners implement the policy.
Health organizations may involve changes in health services and personnel work such as understanding the use of training programmes and quality assurance systems.

Evaluation is usually defined as a method of measuring the extent to which an intervention achieves its stated objectives. However, it should also focus on indicators that relate to efficiency, effectiveness, economy and equity.

'Efficiency' is the extent to which aims and objectives are attained. This can be judged by comparing the results obtained in separate interventions using different methods; or, differing methods used in similar interventions may be compared with each other to see which is achieving the best objectives. Efficiency is sometimes measured by 'good practice' indicators or measures of success.

'Effectiveness' is the extent to which the objectives set have actually led to the desired immediate, intermediate and long-term outcomes. In other words, has the intervention been worthwhile? 'Effectiveness' can also include increased responsiveness to local needs, enhanced team-working, and health and social gains for clients and communities.

'Economy' measures the extent to which all the outcomes (immediate, intermediate, and long-term outcomes) have been achieved economically or may be said to deliver 'value for money'. While costing analysis compares the cost of an intervention to the costs of competing activities, cost-benefit analysis is more complicated and relies on pricing both the inputs (facilities, staff, materials, equipment etc.) and the benefits of the intervention (increased access to services, positive changes in attitude, knowledge and behaviour, reductions in 'risk behaviour' etc.). Putting a price on health and social need outcomes is a very difficult exercise.

'Equity' or 'equality' is the extent to which everyone should ideally have a fair opportunity to attain their full health potential and no one should be disadvantaged from achieving it. However, this does not prescribe equality of outcomes, which would be unrealistic, but merely the availability of equal opportunities and the reduction of barriers to achieving health.

TYPES OF EVALUATION

Øvretveit (1998) describes several major types of evaluation, a number of which are defined below.

- *Needs assessment*   This provides 'baseline' information and a health and social needs profile of a group or community to identify gaps and barriers in service delivery, and issues of access.
- *Project monitoring*   This provides the basic 'building blocks' of evaluation by looking at pilot work, general costings, descriptions of the inputs, activities and outputs. Monitoring may also identify a range of practical difficulties which will need to be understood and overcome.
- *Formative evaluation*   This is a type of 'developmental' evaluation. A formative evaluation focuses on the production of data (usually qualitative measures) in the course of an intervention which can be fed back with the aim of improving it further within its local context.
- *Process evaluation*   This focuses on the 'process' of the evaluation. It may use quantitative or qualitative measures to assess inputs, activities and outputs and to examine how the intervention is organized, delivered and received. Process

evaluation differs from formative evaluation in that it only looks at the process, whereas the latter may also gather information about outcomes. Process evaluation likes to use 'softer' methodologies like participant observation and focus groups. The intention is to assess progress and improve effectiveness by providing an understanding of how the intervention operates and how it produces what it does rather than with assessing long-term effects or outcomes.

- *Implementation evaluation*   These evaluations are concerned with how well or to what extent a treatment, intervention, service or policy was implemented. This is a form of 'audit' evaluation because the evaluation is compared to a model of an intended policy or service. Information is therefore gathered to assess the extent to which the evaluated differs from the intended. This is a type of 'managerial' evaluation.
- *Summative evaluation*   This is aimed at determining the essential effectiveness of interventions and to help decision-makers decide whether to continue an intervention or policy – in other words to 'sum it up'. This style of evaluation involves measuring outputs of performance and outcomes against targets, as well as assessing resources employed. This style of evaluation is usually done for management or for those external to the programme, such as funders, rather than service providers internal to the programme.
- *Outcome or impact evaluation*   This type of evaluation concentrates on discovering the outcomes of an intervention assessed against programme goals and would certainly be part of a summative evaluation, may be part of a formative evaluation but would not be an element in process evaluation.
- *Economic evaluation*   This aims to look at the efficiency of the intervention in terms of the relation between costs and benefits, not only in 'money' terms but also in terms of the improvement in health, the promotion of access and the development of equity. Equity requires that policies and provisions do not in practice affect some people less favourably than others.
- *Pluralistic evaluation*   This style of evaluation investigates the views of different interest groups regarding their definition of success and the extent to which the programme has achieved this. It provides an ethnography of the intervention and an explanation of the processes involved in terms of the interests of participating groups. In addition, it may provide more complex conclusions about the success of the programme on a range of 'value' criteria.

See also Table 5.1 for guide to the focus of different types of evaluation.

CHRONOLOGICAL PHASES IN AN EVALUATION

It must be remembered that each evaluation presents a unique set of circumstances and while evaluation procedures may be applied directly to many situations, it may also be necessary to adapt or modify techniques in order to fit others. At times a creative approach may be required and this is perfectly acceptable. Throughout this handbook certain key terms will be applied to different phases in the progress of the evaluation. Listed below are the main terms as they might appear within the chronology of evaluation (Table 5.2).

Table 5.1 A guide to the focus of different types of evaluation

Pre-evaluation	Evaluation	Post-evaluation

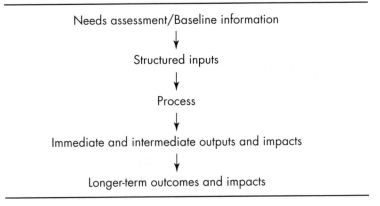

Types of evaluation		
Needs assessment	*Process*	*Impact*
Developmental HIA	Formative Pluralistic Implementation Audit Health impact assessment (HIA) Monitoring	Outcome Summative (HIA)

Table 5.2 Chronological phases in an evaluation

Needs assessment/Baseline information
↓
Structured inputs
↓
Process
↓
Immediate and intermediate outputs and impacts
↓
Longer-term outcomes and impacts

OVERVIEW OF THE KEY TERMS IN THE CHRONOLOGICAL PHASES OF EVALUATION

Needs assessment / baseline information   All evaluations require some form of baseline information or needs assessment to allow achievements to be measured against a 'yardstick' or 'benchmark'. This includes collecting information on the prevalence and nature of the health and social problem or the psychosocial risk indicators such as smoking, poor housing, unemployment, homelessness etc. within the target group or community (see case study, Chapter 10).

Structured inputs   This includes the context of the intervention and the resources necessary to formulate the planned content as well as the staff, knowledge, skills, buildings, equipment and overheads required to undertake the intervention (see case study, Chapter 11).

Process   This is the manner in which the structured inputs are applied to achieve intended outputs and should provide an opportunity for reflection and analysis. The process of an evaluation should give us an insight into the 'illuminative' processes which are involved in programme implementation and the social and environmental context in which they take place (see case study, Chapter 12).

Immediate and intermediate outputs   These are the early impacts of the intervention such as the establishment of advice services, telephone counselling, crèche facilities, housing improvements, empowering individuals and communities etc. Since many of these outputs/impacts can be measured and assessed early in the development of the intervention, we can assess them as immediate outputs/impacts (approximately 3–6 months) and intermediate outputs/impacts (approximately 1 year) and both can provide effective measurement of quality and success (see case study, Chapter 13).

Longer-term outcomes   These are the consequences arising from the outputs/impacts and may take several years for measurement. The outcomes may include an assessment of the impact on inequalities in health as well as improvements in access to services, education and employment.

These terms cover the evaluation style most applicable and best suited to targeting health and social need projects, namely, the pluralistic model and we will now look at its strengths and weaknesses.

PLURALISTIC EVALUATION

Qualitative and quantitative methods

The practice of multidisciplinary teams working in the health field and working across disciplines has led to the call for greater pluralism in attitudes and in the employment of different research evaluative methods. This requires the use of a multi-method approach which recognizes the need to use a mixture of qualitative and quantitative methods. It may be worth remembering basic definitions of these two research methods:

Qualitative methods   this is a form of data collection used to record and understand people's experience and the meanings they give to events and behaviour, e.g. observation techniques, case studies, ethnography, focus groups, content analysis, grounded theory techniques, unstructured interviews.

Quantitative methods   this is a form of data collection whereby the evaluator assigns numbers to an aspect of the person, organization or event and provides measurement tools. These methods are often used within an experimental design which seeks to test hypotheses and includes the randomized control trial, quasi-experimental designs, cohort studies, before-and-after studies, case control studies, structured interviews, questionnaire designs and surveys.

The suggested ideal evaluation methodology proposed for health promotion derived from academic journals is the randomized control trial (RCT). For a long time this classic evaluation design has been seen as the 'proper' evaluation of a treatment or service and has been referred to as the 'gold standard'. The idea behind it is the creation of two groups which are exactly the same in all aspects apart from the fact that one group receives the intervention. One group is called the 'experimental group' and the other the 'control group' and both contain 'subjects'. The 'experiment' tests a hypothesis, not the intervention per se. However, in the area of promoting health, randomized control trials are rare and are perceived to be difficult to undertake to a rigorous scientific standard. The majority of literature from specialist health promotion sources advocates individual, social and environmental perspectives in evaluation and a battery of data collecting and investigative methodologies (Tones and Tilford, 1994; Macdonald, 1996). These authors suggest that it is often difficult to attribute cause and effect from such evaluations and argue that a more 'pluralistic' approach to evaluation is needed, which will incorporate qualitative and quantitative methods.

Much debate centres around the use of qualitative and quantitative methods. The reader of this handbook need not be concerned with the on-going heated debate about the philosophical perspective within which each method is used. It is enough to understand that each method has its rightful place and can produce reliable, valid and objective measures. Although a variety of methods can be used, the implementation of the intervention will often be most appropriately examined using qualitative methods. While quantitative methods can tell us 'how much' and 'how many' or 'to what extent' they tell us very little about 'how' and 'why'. Qualitative methods are particularly useful in process evaluation for answering these questions and identifying user involvement, organizational problems, pitfalls in implementation, stakeholder perceptions of success and barriers to success.

Much evaluation from the quantitative, more experimental, tradition reflects a top-down approach in which interventions are said to be delivered and participants are referred to as 'subjects'. Where there is a stronger commitment to more qualitative methods the relationship between evaluators, organizations and participants is presented differently. Participants are seen as 'collaborators', knowledgeable people with a stake in the utility of the findings. These different partners contribute different dimensions to the evaluation, including technical and research skills, organizational ones, local knowledge and community cohesiveness.

PROCESS EVALUATION

Process evaluation employs a wide range of methods such as semi-structured interviews, focus groups, diaries, taped interviews, participant observation, and content analysis of documents. These methods give a great deal of information about the factors that may be responsible for the intervention's success or failure but they are unable to predict what would happen if it was replicated in other areas (see case study, Chapter 12). Qualitative evaluation gives evidence of appropriateness: the extent to which care can be said to meet the perceived needs of the individual to whom it is offered and evidence of the factors that affect decision-making among policy-makers, clinicians and patients, i.e. why people (lay and professional) behave the way they do. Therefore the multi-faceted aspects of process evaluation need to be built into measures of effectiveness. Macdonald (1996) suggests that

> qualitative research methodology has much to offer in illuminating both process and outcome. Only through this type of research can details be supplied such as 'why' a given programme has or has not achieved its objectives. It can provide details into 'how' outcomes were achieved rather than 'whether' they were achieved. Some researchers argue that the next step is for qualitative research to develop its own hierarchy for quality of method and produce its own 'gold standard'.

This passage illustrates that to understand why some interventions succeed and others fail we need to describe or illuminate what is happening in interventions so that we can make reasoned judgments about what particular features are effective. For this reason we need to use qualitative techniques which provide 'rich description'. However, this does not mean removing the concept of validity as qualitative work can provide very good checks on validity by using 'triangulation', a concept which is described below.

TRIANGULATION AND THE QUESTION OF VALIDITY

The term 'triangulation' derives from the world of surveying where the use of two or more bearings, rather than one, enables a position to be located precisely (Tones, 1994). Similarly, triangulation in the context of evaluation involves accumulating evidence from a variety of sources. If data from an intervention all point in the same direction, it may be reasonable to assume that the programme has been successful and valuable insights have been gained.

For those who wish to find out more about the advantages and main elements of triangulation, these have been emphasized by many authors (Secker, 1995; Macdonald, 1996) and fully explored by Rossi and Freeman (1993), who have identified four main kinds of evidence: data triangulation; investigator triangulation; theory triangulation; and methodological triangulation.

However, bear in mind that a method may give valid data about something, but can be invalid for the evaluation. For instance, a patient's view is valid information about a treatment, but it is invalid information for an evaluation which does not have patients' views as a criterion for value. Following the pathway through the phases will provide answers to the most pertinent initial questions of evaluation. With such definitions and methodologies to assist us we are now ready to embark upon a description of the various steps which make up evaluation.

FURTHER READING

Armstrong, D. and Grace, J. (1994) *Research Methods and Audit in General Practice.* Oxford: Oxford University Press.

Barr, A., Hashagan, S. and Purcell, R. (1996) *Monitoring and Evaluation of Community*

Development in Northern Ireland: a report commissioned by the Voluntary Activity Unit, Department of Health and Social Services. DHSS: Northern Ireland.

Barr, A., Hashagan, S. and Purcell, R. (1996) Measuring Community Development in Northern Ireland – A Handbook for Practitioners. DHSS: Northern Ireland.

Calvert, J., Salmon, S., Lazenbatt, A. and Sinclair, M. (2001) The use of telemedicine to support breastfeeding at home. Journal of Telemedicine and Telecare, 6(1), Suppl. 1:200.

Coup, O. (1990) 'We are doing well, aren't we?' A Guide to Planning, Monitoring and Evaluating Community Projects. Wellington, New Zealand: Department of Internal Affairs.

Funnell, R., Oldfield, K. and Speller,V. (1995) A Tool towards Planning, Evaluating and Developing Healthier Alliances. London: Health Education Authority.

Hawe, P. (1990) Evaluating Health Promotion: A Health Workers Guide. Sydney: McLennan and Petty.

Jones, R. and Kinmouth, A.L. (1995) Critical Reading for Primary Care. Oxford: Oxford University Press.

Lazenbatt, A. (1997) The Contribution of Nurses, Midwives and Health Visitors to Targeting Health and Social Need. Belfast: The Stationery Office.

Lazenbatt, A. McWhirter, L., Bradley, M., and Orr, J. (1999) The role of nursing partnership interventions in improving the health of disadvantaged women. Journal of Advanced Nursing, 30(6): 1280–1288.

Lazenbatt, A., McWhirter, L., Bradley, M., and Orr, J. (2000) Community nursing achievements in targeting health and social need. Nursing Times Research, 5(3): 178–192.

Lazenbatt, A., McWhirter, L., Bradley, M., Orr, J. and Chambers, M. (2000) Tackling inequalities in health and social wellbeing – evidence of 'good practice' by nurses, midwives and health visitors. International Journal of Nursing Practice, 6(2) April: 76–88.

Lazenbatt, A. (2000) Tackling inequalities in health in Northern Ireland. Community Practitioner, 73(2): 481–483.

Lazenbatt, A. and Hunter, P. (2000) 'An evaluation of a drop-in centre for working women'. Queen's University of Belfast/Royal College of Nursing, Northern Ireland.

Lazenbatt, A., Sinclair, M., Salmon, S. and Calvert, J. (2001) Telemedicine as a support system to encourage breastfeeding in Northern Ireland: a case study design. Journal of Telemedicine and Telecare (in press).

Lazenbatt, A. and Orr, J. (2001) Evaluation and effectiveness in practice. International Journal of Nursing Practice, 7(6): (in press).

Lazenbatt, A., Lynch, U. and O'Neill, E. (2001) Revealing the hidden 'troubles' in Northern Ireland: the role of Participatory Rapid Appraisal. Health Education Research (in press).

Macdonald, G. (1996) Where next for evaluation? Health Promotion International, 11: 54–58.

Nutbeam, D. (1993) Evaluation designs in long-term community-based promotion programmes. Journal of Epidemiology and Community Health, 47: 127–133.

Øvretveit, J. (1998) Evaluating health interventions. Buckingham: Open University Press.

Patton, M. Q. (1986) Utilization-focused Evaluation, 2nd edn. London: Sage.

Philips, C., Palfrey, C. and Thomas, P. (1994) Evaluating Health and Social Care. Basingstoke: Macmillan.

Rossi, P. and Freeman, H. (1993) Evaluation: A Systematic Approach. London: Sage.

Secker, J. (1995) Qualitative methods in health promotion research: some criteria for quality. Health Education Journal, 54(1): 74–87.

Sinclair, M. and Lazenbatt, A. (2000) Telesupport in breastfeeding. Computers in Education, special edition, 34: 341–343.

Tones, K. and Tilford, S. (1994) Health Education – Effectiveness, Efficiency and Equity. London: Chapman and Hall.

Voluntary Activity Development Branch (1996) Guidance on the Commissioning and Conduct of Evaluations of Voluntary Organizations by Northern Ireland Government Departments. DHSS: The Stationery Office.

CHAPTER 6

EVALUATING INTERVENTIONS

START THINKING ABOUT THE EVALUATION

Thinking and clarifying the 'who' and 'what' issues involved in evaluation may help people new to evaluation to understand its dimensions. The listings below should not be taken as implying that planning and designing an evaluation is just a matter of answering questions or of following a simple sequence. There is a dynamic between each of the areas and questions listed below. Hopefully it also alerts evaluators of the need to plan how their time will be used and of the need to relate the choices which they make to the resources that are allocated.

Think and clarify:

Who

Who is the evaluation for?

Self-evaluation, local groups, funding/ purchasing body?

Who will be responsibile for the evaluation? Self or an expert in evaluation?
Who will be involved in the evaluation? Organization/practitioner/client group?
Who will be the target group/participants? Is it the whole group or a sub-group?
Whose value perspectives are included? Users helping to focus questions
Who will have access to or own the results? Self, funders, community
Who is the audience receiving the evaluation Language-appropriate format for lay as
report? well as professional groups. Do service providers/managers need feedback?

What

What is being evaluated and why? Main objectives – flexible or rigid?
What method of evaluation will be used? Survey, interviews, observation, questionnaires?

What are the aims and objectives?	Derived from the analysis of the health and social need problem?
What should be measured/recorded?	Process, intermediate or outcome measures or impacts?
What will be the timescale of the evaluation?	Longitudinal or short term?
What resources are allocated to the evaluation?	Limited budget or external funding?
What constitutes success?	Success characteristics?
What are the lessons to be learnt?	Comparison with others/areas to avoid in future evaluations.
What effects upon health and social need?	Impacting or reducing inequalities in health and social need.
Clarify	
Is the evaluation worth the effort?	Is it in-depth or an overview evaluation – expensive?
How will the results be handled?	Qualitatively or quantitatively?
Consideration of alternative explanations?	Anticipate explanations and design evaluation to exclude them.

GETTING STARTED IN EVALUATION

Many evaluations run through a cycle (Figure 6.1), although not necessarily in a precise chronological sequence.

DIFFERENT PHASES OF EVALUATION

Although evaluation is ideally an on-going activity as indicated by its cyclic nature, it nevertheless needs to be divided into chronological phases, as stated previously, which correspond to aspects of the total evaluation, namely:

* Needs assessment (baseline measures)
* Structure (planning phase)
* Process (illumination phase)
* Outcome (review phase).

For purposes of organizational clarity, in the following discussion the various stages of the entire evaluation framework will be classified within these three major phases (see Table 6.1).

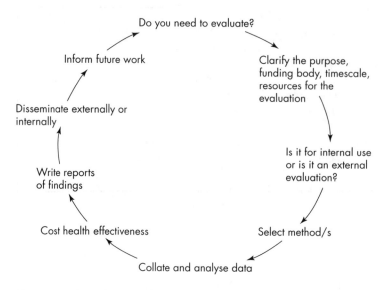

Figure 6.1   The evaluation cycle

Table 6.1 A rough guide to the different phases of an evaluation

Needs	Structure	Process	Outcomes
Baseline Priorities Needs	The amount and quality of:	Activities	Changes in health, attitude, knowledge. Strengthening of individuals and communities
The needs of different: individuals groups sub-populations communities areas	Buildings Equipment Staff Training needs Clients, patients, users	Impact Assessment Intervention Procedures Methods Compliance with 'best' practice	Patient satisfaction Health impacts Psychological / Social outcomes Immediate / Intermediate and longer-term health outcomes

WORKING THROUGH AN EVALUATION

Chapters 7, 8 and 9 each describes one phase of evaluation, within which are several stages. This overall structure is outlined below.

Structure: 'planning' phase

Decide:

- Stage 1: Why are you evaluating?
- Stage 2: Who will be involved in the evaluation?
- Stage 3: When to evaluate? – resources, planning and timescale

Process 'illumination' phase

Decide:

- Stage 4: What information is needed?
- Stage 5: Which measures will be used?
- Stage 6: Which measures suit success indicators of interventions within the area of inequalities?

Outcome 'review' phase

Decide:

- Stage 7: What the measures show? results
- Stage 8: Who should be told? dissemination
- Stage 9: Why review the evaluation?

CHAPTER 7

WORKING THROUGH AN EVALUATION: STRUCTURE

STAGE 1: WHY ARE YOU EVALUATING?

Evaluation is sometimes a complicated and time-consuming process and uses resources which might otherwise be used for programme planning and implementation. How do we justify using scarce resources to evaluate? We evaluate within the area of inequalities in health to improve the quality of an intervention and provide evidence of effectiveness and the contribution that it is making to improving the health and wellbeing of individuals and groups. Below we provide quality guidelines under a number of headings.

Improvements in health and social need

The intervention should:

- impact on poverty and deprivation
- impact on inequalities and inequities in health and social need between the communities in the province
- apply self and community empowerment models of health promotion
- impact on the quality of life of individuals and use a range of measurements and indicators including the qualitative, quantitative and subjective.

Effective delivery of appropriate healthcare

The intervention should:

- develop and clarify indicators of quality and success for a health promoting intervention
- ensure that all objectives have been met and results assessed
- ensure that an intervention is having its intended immediate, intermediate and longer-term outcome effects
- help prevent reinventing the wheel by disseminating the evaluation results to others working in the area and establishing the effectiveness of different methods and strategies.

Fair access

The intervention should ensure that it:

- values and applies needs assessment methods
- identifies factors that are proving barriers to access and change
- helps inform future inequality interventions of problem areas/weaknesses, including how accessible and user-friendly they are and how they build on the knowledge base
- accommodates the complex interactivity of individuals involved in the evaluation from practitioners, funders, managers, to organizations and users – this process allows everyone's voice to be heard.

Efficiency

The intervention should ensure that it:

- assists in understanding the relative costs/benefits of different models of programme/service provision and so contributes to effective targeting of services;
- espouses organizational, practitioner and user involvement in the planning and delivery of healthcare programmes.

STAGE 2:   WHO SHOULD BE INVOLVED IN THE EVALUATION?

Different stakeholders

Success and quality mean different things to different groups of people or 'stakeholders'. Any form of evaluation must take into account the varying needs and perceptions of all people involved, since they will be investing alternative interests or looking for different results in an intervention. Whenever possible this should include the involvement of user groups, clients, patients and other community members in designing and carrying out evaluations, in analysing the results and in planning changes to the intervention.

We can evaluate an item on behalf of one or more of the following perspectives or interest groups: patients, clients, lay workers, users; health and social care practitioners; managers; politicians; health researchers; the media.

Implementation of the results of an evaluation is more likely if the evaluation has paid attention to the concerns and questions of interest groups which can support or oppose changes.

A number of phrases are commonly used in the definition of expectations by stakeholders:

- the 'quality' of the intervention is the degree to which it meets the requirements of its stakeholders (sponsors, practitioners, clients, managers)

- the 'effectiveness' of an intervention is the extent to which it meets the needs of its users (clients)
- the 'efficiency' of an intervention measures the resources it consumes in relation to its effectiveness (sponsors, managers, policy-makers)
- 'value for money' is an aspiration concerned with achieving maximal efficiency, meeting all the quality criteria at minimal cost (managers, sponsors, practitioners).

Working in partnership

An acknowledgement should be made that all investing parties are involved in an evaluation. Data should be collected from each group or stakeholder and as defined earlier this is referred to as Pluralistic Evaluation. Health and wellbeing is not given by providers to an individual or a community, rather health and social wellbeing is promoted through partnerships that involve collaborative working relationships and meaningful interactions between health and social care providers and the community.

A variety of terms are used to describe these interactions, such as networks, partnerships, collaborations, alliances, coalitions, cooperatives, affiliations, multidisciplinary teams, joint ventures, mergers, clinical teams.

The term 'collaboration' means 'working together'; thus partnerships may comprise two or more organizations working together on a community issue, or multidisciplinary teams and voluntary agencies working together in the clinical field. Partnerships must be flexible and built on the unique contributions that each partner brings to the situation such as benefits derived from extending the range of skills, experiences and perspectives available. Because every situation demands different contributions from each partner, the distribution of power in the partnership also needs to be negotiated. Effective negotiating requires self–other awareness, flexibility and sometimes mediation.

Partnerships must evolve in their structure and effectiveness with a mutual goal to strengthen and empower individuals or the community. In this case the goal is to enable an individual or community to assume responsibility for their/its health first by understanding issues, thinking through possible solutions and finally by making informed decisions that will impact. Each partner will produce data and, by using triangulation techniques which employ a wide range of data sources, an overall picture can be built up, which is more complex, more complete and more valid. In this respect evaluation should be seen as a bridge linking practitioners, health promoters and others such as funders, clients, users and organizations (private/statutory and voluntary).

The organization and establishment of a partnership

The process often starts with providers attempting to assess an individual's or community's needs or its degree of satisfaction with access to existing healthcare services. In building a partnership the organizational phase lays the foundation for the main activities of the intervention. It is crucial that organizers gain active and passive support from patients, clients, local groups and community stakeholders. With encouragement and effective facilitation, informal discussions among individuals can evolve into a structured community–provider partnership. However, there can be a number of barriers to effective client/community/provider partnering and these are listed below.

- Suspicion of new activities (either partner)
- Lack of information about the need for change
- History of conflict among key community members
- History of competition among stakeholders
- Lack of vision and visibility by organizers of partnership
- Frequent change of administration in partnership
- Resistance to outside influence by the community
- Negative experiences with past partnering efforts (either partner)
- Threat of losing intervention (usually providers)
- Trust violations (usually providers).

There are various criteria for including the input of an organization in an evaluation. It may be necessary to know if they provide a systematic data collection which illustrates within a locality the extent of poverty, deprivation, access to services, gender, age, occupation, social class of its population. Also, ascertain whether they have information about health, social conditions and the use of services in local areas which is easy to read and understand and is based on data collection. In terms of their own organization, it may be worth looking at their aims and objectives and any public declaration to reduce inequalities in health. Do they have inequality strategies which encompass all partner organizations and their departments and which reflect the needs of different groups, e.g. women, men, children, the elderly, ethnic minorities, travellers, the homeless, lone parents, and the disabled? Finally, it is worth knowing if they have systematic funding for community health issues using a community development model; and are involved in training of service providers to raise their awareness of inequalities and to improve the quality of response to people within this area.

The client/user and the establishment of a partnership

To be successful and to make meaningful progress an intervention should take a greater account of the views of people whose health and social wellbeing it seeks to improve. To do this an evaluation requires participation in decision-making by local people, with co-operation between lay people and professionals. This may entail establishing effective local alliances across professional and organizational boundaries, with co-operation between and within departments and agencies.

Evaluation focusing on the user perspective should cover issues such as the individual's:

- concepts of holistic health, ill health, positive health, psychological health, social health, disability and handicap
- subjective views of health
- knowledge of, use of, evaluation and perceived integration of available services
- desired changes in services and accessibility of services
- priorities for the use of scarce resources
- views of the needs of people who do not use existing services.

Another advantage of learning more about user perspectives is that they can provide a more holistic picture of systems of care. People seeking help with health and social problems often feel exposed to a bewildering array of services and organizations. Evaluation of the user perspective cannot begin to be useful unless the findings fully, accurately and sensitively reflect their beliefs, feelings, and aspirations. An adequate methodology for investigating users' perspectives requires that the right people are asked the right questions, that they answer in ways that reflect their true beliefs and feelings and that their answers are interpreted correctly. In order to select the client/user group the evaluator should define the population of theoretical interest; identify its interest; gain access to and persuade them to participate in the evaluation; and question them in user-friendly language.

The Box contains a number of questions that you can check to assist you in deciding who should be included in the evaluation.

Who will be involved in the evaluation?

Working alone or in a group check the questions below to decide who should be involved in an intervention

Participants

- Will members of the target group be involved in the design and development of the intervention?
- Will the target groups' needs be assessed appropriately to shape the intervention?
- Will the setting be accessible and accepted by the target audience?
- How homogeneous is the population of interest, e.g. would it be more appropriate to deliver the intervention to individuals or groups, rural/urban mix?
- Will the intervention reduce barriers between different groups?
- Will it improve communication between all parties?
- Will the context of the intervention be educationally and culturally appropriate to the target group?
- Will the intervention be flexibly delivered?
- Will adequate outreach into the community take place to identify which parties/ groups need to be included?

Measuring user/client/consumer effects

Working alone or in a group check the questions below to decide issues in the measurement of client/user/consumer effects

- Will the initiative *change* attitudes and behaviour as well as increasing knowledge?
- Will users' opinions be *sought* on issues relating to health?

- Will surveys, telephone interviews, focus groups etc. be used to assess satisfaction, attitudes, knowledge and behaviour?
- Will users be involved in *decision-making* about their health?
- Will users be involved in *influencing policy*?
- Will there be the development of *empowerment* for individuals, groups and communities?
- Will health and social *gains be measured* for the client group?
- Will users be involved in the *process* of evaluation?

Who will be doing the evaluation?

Selecting the right person to carry out the evaluation is crucial. Will this be the project worker, researcher or someone from an outside agency/organization or a combination of both? Remember to be clear about objectivity and consider that local people or lay health workers can be involved in the evaluation and trained to carry out data collections and benefit from being paid and employed while gaining qualifications (see case study, Chapter 10). Collaboration and working in multidisciplinary teams can bring together people with a range of skills and experiences. All staff involved should agree who will conduct the evaluation.

The person undertaking the evaluation needs to understand the interests of the different stakeholder groups and how they may be affected by the on-going evaluation and its findings. Evaluators and users need to think ahead to the possible practical implications of different findings. They need to understand who will gain, lose, be hurt or harmed by these types of findings. It is best to take practical and technical issues and ethical obligations into consideration at the planning stage of evaluation to consider the impact of the evaluation. Øvretveit (1998) suggests consideration should also be directed to the four key areas outlined below.

Trust and credibility   When conducting an evaluation the evaluator should be perceived as a trusted, impartial professional who 'speaks the language' of all those involved. Establishing trust and credibility is essential to a successful evaluation. Trust takes time to establish and is the result of an evaluator balancing honesty and discretion. Credibility comes from proving one's competence and also from pointing out the limitations of this competence.

Access and cooperation   Politics and motives can affect how easy it is for an evaluator to gain access to and cooperation from personnel, clients and patients. Gaining access requires negotiating skills as well as persistence and the person should be seen as someone who understands the practical problems and is prepared to be flexible in arranging interviews and other methods of data collection.

Hidden agendas   There are many different reasons why funders and others want to evaluate and sometimes there are 'hidden' reasons such as delay tactics or political reasons. Evaluators should always aim to stay unaware of these issues as they could bias the data collection or findings.

Confidentiality   Issues regarding confidentiality always arise in an evaluation. It is essential, when negotiating access to patient/client records and documents that are not in the public domain, that an evaluator ensures that agreement is made as to what information can and cannot be reported in published reports and materials. When conducting interviews and using questionnaires all evaluators need to state the code of confidentiality which applies to these methods of collecting data.

Checklist of questions to assess who will do the evaluation

- *Who will conduct the evaluation?*   Independent evaluator, project worker, team collaboration, health practitioner. Has a similar evaluation been undertaken elsewhere and can this be accessed and used?
- *Who will be in the evaluation team?*   Does the evaluation team have the necessary required skills and knowledge of:
    - questionnaire design
    - statistical expertise
    - health economics
    - qualitative methods
    - health impact assessment
    - ways of reducing inequalities in health.
    - Do you need to seek outside help and what type of help would compliment in-house skills?
- *Who will be the lead person?*   Member of the team/collaboration or will there be more than one lead person?
- *Will the delivery agent require evaluation training?*   Will this be in-house or require specific training?
- *Will the community/individual/user require training?*   In-house, volunteer, peer education/support training?
- *What other resources are needed for the person to do the work?*   Extra staff, equipment, time, stationery, clerical skills etc.
- *How can the cost be reduced?*   Can expertise and resources be gained through collaborating with other agencies or by building alliances?
- *What detail and accuracy of information does the person need to collect?*   Standardized questionnaires, coding and data analysis expertise?
- *Will they need to be aware of data protection, confidentiality and the ethics of the intervention?*   Ethics committees and community forums?

STAGE 3: WHEN TO EVALUATE

Resources

It is important to establish a clear view of what the costs (inputs) and benefits (outputs) of any intervention may be. All interventions assessing health and social need require some form of cost-analysis or evidence of effectiveness. Most people when they talk of 'cost' usually think in economic or monetary terms, however, 'costs' refer to all types of inputs such as the context of the intervention (the premises), the planned content, the number of staff, their skills and training needs, knowledge input, budgets, equipment and buildings etc. Benefits on the other are consequences arising from the outputs, e.g. more people claiming benefits, less people smoking, reduced teenage pregnancies, less accidents in the home, improved childcare facilities, housing conditions improved, increased employment etc. Economic evaluation does not have the objective of improving the quality of life 'at lowest cost', rather it is concerned with efficiency, i.e. the relation between benefits and costs, and should be seen as providing a set of techniques for the identification and measurement of efficiency.

The most important concept in economic evaluation is that of 'Opportunity costs'. This refers to the value of the work that is presently on-going because you are investing time and money in this work. By comparing the value of what is forfeited with the benefits of what is now supported, it is possible to decide whether the new intervention provides value for money. Another important concept is 'Marginal cost'. This refers to any extra cost, e.g. extra home visits/medical staff, accommodation, clerical assistance, equipment etc.

Ten questions about resources to consider before embarking on an evaluation

- Why is the evaluation being undertaken?   *Opportunity costs*
- Who will lead the evaluation?   *Labour costs*
- Who will do the work?   *Labour costs*
- Has a similar evaluation been undertaken elsewhere and can this be accessed and reviewed?   *Reduced labour costs*
- Are the skills present in the intervention to lead and undertake the work? *Training costs*
- Should outside help be sought and what type of help would complement in-house skills?   *Consultancy costs*
- What other resources are needed to do the evaluation?   *Capital investments costs (new premises, equipment etc.) or fixed costs*
- How can the cost of the evaluation be minimized?   *Marginal costs*
- What detail and accuracy of information is needed?   *Labour costs*
- Are data protection and confidentiality likely to be relevant in this evaluation? *Time and labour costs*

Remember that it is most important that you stipulate where the money will go by measuring the resource use (i.e. costs) and relating it back to baseline measures (this is information that you should have collected at the beginning of any intervention). Unless this is done you have no yardstick to measure your achievements or ways of assessing what changes have occurred. You will then be able to calculate the evaluation's success in meeting its stated objectives. Consult a health economist as there are a number of formal methods for amalgamating costs and benefits into a single ratio with techniques such as cost-effectiveness and cost-utility analysis. However, a sufficient and useful method is the cost consequence analysis. This can be done by specifying the cost of your evaluation and separately identifying outcome gains and losses.

The results might show that the intervention was a resounding success or they may show areas that have gained and others which have made only a limited difference, e.g. staff satisfaction with the intervention may have increased while the user perspective may have decreased. This method allows you to observe the range of effects and enables you and your collaborators to decide upon the strengths or weaknesses of the intervention. However, evaluation is never without costs.

Planning your evaluation costs

- Select baseline costing information
- Labour costs – staff, data collectors, secretarial, clerical, multidisciplinary teams, other agencies (count people as well as an activity)
- Non-labour costs – equipment, premises, transport, computers, consumables, administration, postage etc., equipment hire, travel costs
- Think of indirect costs: team members' time, use of clinic, health service facility, community facility etc., e.g. rooms, telephone, electricity, heat etc.
- Costing of data collections – in-house information systems can provide costings
- Researcher's fees (£250 a day for university-based consultancy)
- Report production – dissemination process
- Printing and stationery
- Decide on bottom-up or top-down costings.

Overall, are there sufficient structural, human and financial resources?

The listings above cover most areas of costing, but are not exhaustive. Bear in mind that sometimes there are hidden costs requiring additional funding. In the total process of costing, you should attempt as far as possible to minimize costs by drawing on relatively inexpensive data, knowledge and skills. It is necessary, of course, to estimate in advance the appropriateness of these to your particular evaluation (see Chapter 11, case study: Setting-up a drop-in centre for prostitutes: a woman centred multi-agency approach).

It is also worth considering resources in terms of knowledge and skills that may be obtained free. These may include literature reviews and critical appraisals (available from librarians or academic units). Libraries and research units can also be used to find evidence-based material, perhaps with the help of search facilities. More broadly, access to Census data, Government Surveys, National and Regional R&D Offices may prove useful.

Resources within the community may include support networks, premises, volunteers for data collections, lay health workers etc. Local information networks can be used, with a lay perspective providing a more holistic picture. Community and locality profiling reports may provide invaluable information.

Decide on the scale of your evaluation, on what support is available and whether or not you need additional resources. Some networks may not be able to offer financial support but can provide instead invaluable methodological expertise, one-to-one support, training etc. Possible contacts for resources and support with collaborations are listed below.

- Statutory funding from central government, e.g. DoH, Department of Health and Social Services, local boards and trusts – particularly commissioning departments, public health medicine and the Health Promotion Agency
- NHS Research and Development Office and regional research and development offices
- Universities and academic research units: schools of nursing, psychology, medicine, dentistry, economics, social policy etc., health service research units, health promotion units
- Medical audit groups and Primary Care Development Fund
- Voluntary organizations, European Social Fund, community networks, consumer networks, fund-raising groups and charities
- Research Councils, e.g. Medical Research Council (MRC), Economic and Social Research Council (ESRC); the Rowntree Foundation, the Wellcome Trust, Leverhulme Trust, Smyth and Nephew
- Private sector and pharmaceutical companies.

Planning and timescale

There is no one way to plan and make an evaluation. Targeting Health and Social Need interventions and programmes, for example, all have different timescales, budgets, and evaluator skills and because of this different effects may become apparent at different time intervals. The assessment of the overall success or failure of an intervention will therefore depend on the timing of the evaluation. As the effects of an intervention may not be apparent for some time, evaluation should always be built in at the beginning of an intervention to allow it to become an integral part of the project. Many evaluations follow a sequence of phases and cover a structure, process and outcome phase (see case study, Chapter 11).

It is important to pilot your work and establish baseline information to allow you to provide a yardstick to measure your achievements against. The initial measures and recordings at the beginning of the evaluation should include baseline information from all stakeholders and needs assessment of a locality or patient group to provide a way of measuring what changes have happened or indeed, by how much (see case study, Chapter 10).

Plan your timescale at the outset. Give yourself enough time, as evaluation always takes longer than you think. Enough time needs to be allocated to assess all the following:

Baseline information, needs assessment	(Time 0)
Process evaluation	(Time 2)
Immediate effects/impacts	(Time 3)
Intermediate outcome	(Time 4)
Long-term outcome effects/impacts	(Time 5)

For example, if the desired outcome is behaviour change, there will be intermediate effects such as changes in knowledge and attitude long before behavioural change itself is seen. A formative style of evaluation should always be considered where rapid feedback about progress is required with supporting analysis and recommendations from the evaluators. The rationale should describe the background to the intervention, the reasons why it has developed and the questions that the evaluation seeks to answer. It is important at this stage to seek out any relevant evaluations that have already been undertaken which suggest an approach likely to produce benefits in terms of achieving health gain, improving quality, cost-effectiveness or other relevant issues. Where there is no such evidence an extensive literature search should be arranged (help with this may be available from university libraries, research units and information specialists).

Setting aims and objectives is very important and they should be stated explicitly. Aims are more general statements that summarize the purpose of the intervention, while objectives are the desired outcomes. Remember that these outcomes depend on a timescale and can range from immediate, intermediate to longer-term outcomes.

By this time you should have formulated a plan which describes (for assessing a completed evaluation substitute the past tense):

- review evidence of best practice in the area
- who the evaluation is for
- who will pay
- a time plan of activities and milestones
- the resources to be used and the budget
- constraints – time frame, resources and expertise
- the purpose of the evaluation, and the one or more questions it aims to answer. Set objectives for the intervention – these should be:
  Specific
  Measurable
  Achievable
  Realistic
  Timely They all add up (SMART!)
- what is to be evaluated
- the evaluation design
- the methods used to gather and analyse data
- impacts/outcomes at all time intervals
- the reporting and dissemination process.

FURTHER READING

Stages 1 and 2

Blaxter, M. (1993) *Consumer Issues within the NHS*. London: Department of Health.

Blaxter, M. (1997) Whose fault is it? People's own conceptions of the reasons for inequalities in health. *Social Science and Medicine*, 44(6): 747–756.

Funnell, V. (1995) *Towards Healthier Alliances: A Tool for Planning and Evaluating*. London: Wessex Public Health Medicine.

Hawe, P. (1995) *Evaluating Health Promotion: a Healthy Workers Guide*. Sydney: MacLennan.

Heyman, R. (1995) *Researching User Perspectives on Community Health Care*. London: Chapman and Hall.

Lazenbatt, A. (2000) Tackling inequalities in health in Northern Ireland. *Community Practitioner*, 73(2): 481–483.

Lazenbatt, A. and Hunter, P. (2000) 'An evaluation of a drop-in centre for working women'. Queen's University of Belfast/Royal College of Nursing, Northern Ireland.

Lazenbatt, A. and Orr, J. (2001) Evaluation and effectiveness in practice. *International Journal of Nursing Practice*, 7(6) (in press).

Lazenbatt, A., McWhirter, L., Bradley, M., and Orr, J. (1999) The role of nursing partnership interventions in improving the health of disadvantaged women. *Journal of Advanced Nursing*, 30(6), 1280–1288.

Lazenbatt, A., McWhirter, L., Bradley, M. and Orr, J. (2000) Community nursing achievements in targeting health and social need. *Nursing Times Research*, 5(3): 178–192.

Lazenbatt, A., McWhirter, L., Bradley, M. Orr, J. and Chambers, M. (2000) Tackling inequalities in health and social wellbeing – evidence of 'good practice' by nurses, midwives and health visitors. *International Journal of Nursing Practice*, 6(2) April: 76–88.

Lazenbatt, A., Sinclair, M., Salmon, S. and Calvert, J. (2001) Telemedicine as a support system to encourage breastfeeding in Northern Ireland: a case study design. *Journal of Telemedicine and Telecare* (in press).

Lazenbatt, A., Lynch, U. and O'Neill, E. (2001) Revealing the hidden 'troubles' in Northern Ireland: the role of Participatory Rapid Appraisal. *Health Education Research* (in press).

McIver, S. (1993) *Obtaining the Views of Users of Primary and Community Health Care Services*. London: King's Fund.

Øvretveit, J. (1998) *Evaluating Health Interventions*. Buckingham: Open University Press.

Voluntary Activity Development Branch (1996) *Guidance on the Commissioning and Conduct of Evaluations of Voluntary Organizations by Northern Ireland Government Departments*. DHSS: The Stationery Office.

Stage 3

Charities Aid Foundation (1995) *Directory of Grant Making Trusts*. London: Villemur.

Clarke, S. (1992) *The Complete Fund-raising Book and Directory of Social Change*. London: ICMF.

Directory of Social Change (1990) *The Central Governments Grant Guide*: London.

Drummond, M., Stoddard, G. and Torrance, G. (1987) *Methods for the Economic Evaluation of Health Care Programmes*. Oxford: Oxford University Press.

Frazer, E. (1995) Evaluating health promotion – doing it by numbers. *Health Education Journal*, 54(2): 214–225.

King, J., Morris, J.N. and Fitz-Gibbon, C. (1988) *How to Assess Programme Implementation*. Newbury Park: Sage.

Kirkbusch, I. (1986) Issues in health promotion. *Health Promotion International*, 1: 437–442.

Lazenbatt, A. (1999) *Manual for Evaluation and Effectiveness in Practice, Volume 2*. Belfast: The Stationery Office.

Lazenbatt, A. (2000) Tackling inequalities in health in Northern Ireland. *Community Practitioner*, 73(2): 481–483.

Lazenbatt, A. and Hunter, P. (2000) 'An evaluation of a drop-in centre for working women'. Queen's University of Belfast/Royal College of Nursing, Northern Ireland.

Lazenbatt, A. and Orr, J. (2001) Evaluation and effectiveness in practice. *International Journal of Nursing Practice*, 7(6) (in press).

Lazenbatt, A., McWhirter, L., Bradley, M. and Orr, J. (1999) The role of nursing partnership interventions in improving the health of disadvantaged women. *Journal of Advanced Nursing*, 30(6): 1280–1288.

Lazenbatt, A., McWhirter, L., Bradley, M. and Orr, J. (2000a) Community nursing achievements in targeting health and social need. *Nursing Times Research*, 5(3): 178–192.

Lazenbatt, A., McWhirter, L., Bradley, M., Orr, J. and Chambers, M. (2000b) Tackling inequalities in health and social wellbeing – evidence of 'good practice' by nurses, midwives and health visitors. *International Journal of Nursing Practice*, 6(2) April: 76–88.

Lazenbatt, A., Sinclair, M., Salmon, S. and Calvert, J. (2001a) Telemedicine as a support system to encourage breastfeeding in Northern Ireland: a case study design. *Journal of Telemedicine and Telecare* (in press).

Lazenbatt, A., Lynch, U. and O'Neill, E. (2001b) Revealing the hidden 'troubles' in Northern Ireland: the role of Participatory Rapid Appraisal. *Health Education Research* (in press).

National Council for Voluntary Organizations (1993) *Finding Funds*, 2nd edn. Oxford: Oxford University Press.

Nutbeam, D. and Wise, M. (1996) Planning for health for all: an international experience in setting health goals and targets. *Health Promotion International*, 11(3): 219–226.

Salter, B. (1993) The politics of purchasing in the NHS. *Policy and Politics*, 21: 171–184.

Tones, K. and Tilford, S. (1994) *Health Education: Effectiveness, Efficiency and Equity*. London: Chapman and Hall.

CHAPTER 8

WORKING THROUGH AN EVALUATION: PROCESS

STAGE 4: WHAT INFORMATION IS NEEDED?

Reviewing knowledge: Evidence of quality or 'best practice'

This is one of the tasks that should take place in the early stages of evaluation. The purpose is to find out what is already known about the evaluated, and to see if or how others have made similar evaluations. In most cases this will take the form of a review of scientific and published literature, and it will also entail finding out if there are any relevant internal documents which have described or reported the evaluated and producing a review of these. This is the time when you want to know what will give you evidence of 'best practice' in healthcare. What then *is* evidence-based healthcare?

We described in Chapter 3 that a commitment to evidence-based healthcare means a commitment to:

- planning to include the needs of the target group and to employ the best of current knowledge as to how to meet these needs
- finding out the effectiveness of that intervention, in other words, who has benefited from it and who has not.

We also cited three sources of evidence of 'best practice' within the area of reducing inequalities in health. These were the findings from the Targeting Health and Social Need (THSN) Project in Northern Ireland (Lazenbatt, 1997a; 2000); the Dutch review by Gepkens and Gunning-Schepers (1995); and the systematic review of interventions to reduce inequalities in health undertaken by researchers at the University of York (see Table 3.1). In the future health professionals should be able to define the criteria by which they can label their interventions as examples of 'best practice' and be able to apply these criteria to all interventions. By combining the results of these three sources of evidence we can highlight 16 characteristics or indicators which can be labeled as criteria by which to judge an intervention as more likely to achieve its aim of impacting upon inequalities in health.

'Best practice'

We have taken 16 success characteristics, which may be used by potential evaluators to decide what importance to attribute to each, and have divided these into four core areas:

- *Approaches/partnerships*   This focuses on collaborations, health alliances, inter-agency working, multidisciplinary team-working, multi-faceted and intensive approaches
- *Tools (methods)*   This focuses on tools such as audit and evaluation, and methods such as research-based needs assessment and health impact assessments
- *Resources*   This focuses on the resources required such as use of support materials, the setting, the importance of and training of the delivery agent
- *Individual/community*   This focuses on the individual/patient or community view of health with elements such as holistic health, culture, community development and empowerment.

These characteristics provide a basis for debating quality measures within inequalities evaluations. It must be stressed, however, that such indicators are not mutually exclusive, nor are the characteristics offered to be taken as exhaustive. It would be unrealistic to think that all inequality interventions would contain all of these indicators. However, it might prove useful to discuss the advantages to the intervention of including those indicators that correctly match the style of intervention that you are evaluating.

The following discussion will define and highlight the characteristics within the four core areas and describe the type of evaluation work that is providing evidence of

Table 8.1 Success indicators

Success indicators	Structure	Process	Outcome
1 Approaches/partnerships			
Health Alliances			
Inter-agency			
Multidisciplinary			
Multifaceted			
2 Tools (methods)			
Audit			
Evaluation			
Research			
Needs assessment			
3 Resources			
Support material			
Setting			
Delivery agent			
Training delivery agent			
4 Individual/community			
Holistic health			
Culture			
Community development			
Empowerment			

success. All of the above areas would fit into one or other of the three areas of activity on which clinical governance and quality assurance processes focus, i.e. structure, processes and outcomes. It might be helpful to select the most appropriate success indicators for your particular evaluation from those listed in Table 8.1 by ticking the relevant boxes. This will give you an overview of 'best practice' indicators through every stage of the evaluation and should prove valuable in the overall planning.

POTENTIAL INDICATORS OR CHARACTERISTICS OF A SUCCESSFUL INEQUALITY INTERVENTION

1   APPROACHES/PARTNERSHIPS

An intensive approach   Vigorous or intensive approaches have been shown to improve the identification and subsequent effective treatment of individuals, particularly those from deprived communities. These intensive programmes involve health professionals and inter-agency alliances tackling a wide range of health and social problems with the aid of community health workers to screen, counsel, follow-up and monitor people with, for example, high blood pressure, alongside smoking and obesity issues, all within a primary care setting. Similar work is on-going in schools with health professionals and teachers working with asthmatic children by illustrating the effects of smoking and pollution and by training teachers about these young people's health needs.

Multifaceted approaches   Successful programmes appear to employ a combination of interventions to improve the health of deprived individuals/communities, e.g. intensive 'stepped care' for those with hypertension. This involves specialist treatment combined with attempts to improve access to the service. Research suggests that combining education and legislation is more effective than education alone, e.g. in modifying children's behaviour in relation to bicycle helmet use.

Partnerships/health alliances/inter-agency working   Successful interventions allow individuals, community groups, inter-agency alliances and voluntary groups to work together with the statutory services to promote health and raise the issues concerned with inequalities. All stakeholders need to share the responsibility of promoting health. Working together has a central part to play in allowing community or layman/user participation into practice. All of these social networks may be an important resource in the process of enabling and empowering people to increase control over or improve their health and social wellbeing. Partnerships can also include the use of peer education, support and self-help groups where help comes from individuals working together.

Multidisciplinary team-working   Working in teams is necessary as no single profession has a monopoly on health or indeed is equipped to resolve multifaceted health issues. There is now a need for new ways of working that involve the creation of supportive health environments to promote collaborative working and provide input from many specialist areas. Multidisciplinary teams or agencies facilitate the adoption of different strategies, the development of improved information systems and the harnessing of resources.

Example: Community Health Information Project (CHIP)

An intensive approach   The Community Health Information Project (CHIP) aims to create a core group of local people with a wealth of knowledge and skills on health and social issues. The skills, acquired through capacity building and training programmes, enable local people to plan and implement a range of health programmes, sensitive to community needs and capacities. The programmes are designed to maintain and improve individual and community health status and wellbeing, as well as shifting the emphasis to 'a person-centred approach'. The person, and by extension the community, having taken ownership of their health needs, are further empowered to influence at central government, regional and local levels the delivery of community health strategies to improve health.

Multifaceted approaches   The aim is to increase the level of accurate and relevant health information available to the community as well as to initiate education and training programmes creating a core group of local people with relevant knowledge and skills to deliver a range of health programmes meeting community needs. The objectives are to:

- develop a wealth of knowledge on a range of health issues which can be shared by others in the community
- dispel myths surrounding health and illness
- identify relevant health issues impacting on the community
- carry out educational and health awareness programmes
- identify a core group of local people to deliver a range of health programmes
- provide appropriate training and support for core group members
- build confidence in local people
- develop further links between health and social services, other relevant agencies and CHIP
- play a co-ordinating role in the development of more formal networking
- develop partnerships between statutory providers, the community and voluntary sector and local people.

Partnerships/health alliances/inter-agency working   The concept of partnership is central to the development of local community health strategies and forms the underlying basis of the project. CHIP was formed following discussions between community unit management and staff, health visitors (public health), health visitors (family), day centre and health centre management and staff, community psychiatric team, community addiction team, educational welfare officers, youth workers, Women's

Aid, NEXUS, Family Planning Association, Community Initiatives, Parent and Toddler Association, and local residents. Core membership is currently 150 members providing a unique blend of individuals with a wide range of expertise. Members with a background in health are able to put their knowledge and expertise to good effect providing training and support for local residents.

Multidisciplinary team-working   Multidisciplinary teams of nurses, midwives, health visitors, dentists, doctors, social workers, psychologists, administration staff and users all work together to provide:

- information evenings, e.g. on alcohol, drug and solvent abuse
- stress management courses
- communication skills courses
- community health festivals
- information leaflets and poster campaigns
- 'Activate' health programmes
- group work skills courses
- round-table meetings with statutory bodies and local people
- child abuse conferences
- joint working party to develop neighbourhood youth projects
- a series of joint meetings to set up 'Community Mother Network'
- joint working party meetings to develop and implement a health survey.

Characteristics of good practice in the Community Health Information Project (CHIP)

- decisions based on needs assessment through local surveys
- allowing local people to assess their own needs for health
- focus on issues affecting holistic health of all age groups
- research-based project
- records the thoughts and ideas of local residents
- increases a sense of achievement of what the community can themselves positively change through increasing 'ownership' of the process
- encourage the local residents and community groups to focus and integrate their energies towards goals which improve the health and social wellbeing of the whole community
- Management Committee drawn from local people, statutory representatives and local community and voluntary agencies
- working in partnerships between professionals and local communities
- positive community development approach
- planned approach to working with and training the community
- team-working with shared goals and objectives

- offering employment
- reducing inequalities in health and social need
- empowering and facilitating local people
- reducing stress and providing 'ways of coping'
- networking and disseminating results
- monitoring and report writing
- evaluation framework using qualitative and quantitative methods.

2   TOOLS (METHODS)

Research-based approach   This is the generation of new knowledge and new approaches which have a general application to the health and wellbeing of both individuals and communities. Evidence is required not only from research but also information about patterns of care, population needs, and the availability of resources to increase the knowledge base about effectiveness, health and environmental impacts and cost-effectiveness. It is essential to know what works and what is ineffective and also there is a need to generate theoretical principles that can be applied to situations and individuals.

Use of previous audit   This is using systematic methods for improving and/or ensuring that the intervention or project meets the needs of local people. Audit is concerned with judging whether an intervention is working effectively in practice and in further assessing whether or not resources are being used to the best advantage. Findings of an audit relate to the work of the team, organization, alliance, partnership or programme. Clinical audit provides a framework within which clinical guidelines, needs assessment, evidence of effectiveness and information on cost-effectiveness can be brought together to improve the quality of patient/client/user care.

Use of previous evaluation   Evaluation and health impact assessment can combine the use of qualitative (interviews, observation, case studies etc.) and quantitative (surveys, questionnaires, RCTs, experimental work etc.) methods.

Prior needs assessment   This is working to find out target group or community health needs profiling to inform a population view of health and social need and to identify gaps in service and barriers to service delivery. Profiling and monitoring the impact of poverty, social exclusion, and deprivation is essential in any evaluation as it produces a baseline measure. Without such information on local deprivation levels and the health and social costs of poverty for individuals and families, evaluators are unlikely to be able to evaluate the effectiveness of current strategies or make judgments about how they should be responding to poverty and health issues.

Example: early detection and effective treatment of postnatal depression

Research-based approach   For the past nine years in this locality health visitors have linked with GPs and mental health teams to improve practice in the detection and management of postnatal depression (PND). Since then health visitors have been using the Edinburgh Postnatal Screening tool, at six to eight weeks following delivery, to identify those mothers who are likely to be suffering from postnatal depression. There is considerable evidence that non-directive counselling or listening therapy by health visitors is helpful to at least two-thirds of mothers suffering from postnatal depression. Those women identified as suffering from postnatal depression are offered an agreed contract of non-directive counselling visits. Non-directive counselling is also known as 'person-centred' therapy because this approach locates power in the client, rather than in the counsellor. The major assumption is that by talking through their feelings with a warm and interested, but non-interfering other person, clients will gradually come to know themselves better, and find solutions to their problems. It is assumed that health visitors already act as counsellors in many situations; however, being non-directive may involve a change in emphasis.

Use of previous audit   Following an audit by the Health Visiting Service in 1995, a multi-professional group including a consultant psychiatrist, midwives (community and acute), a GP, a GP audit facilitator, health visitors, a consultant obstetrician, users of the service (newly delivered mothers) defined a protocol to assist practitioners to detect postnatal depression at an early stage and manage those suffering from it more effectively. The aim of the intervention was to screen all mothers in their homes 6–8 weeks following delivery using the Edinburgh Postnatal Depression Scale.

Use of previous evaluation   Evaluation of the programme has shown:

- a high level of expertise and skill by GPs, health visitors and midwives in identifying and managing PND which illustrates the benefits of multidisciplinary working
- an awareness and significance of this distressing illness to the local community. It allows screening to be 'normalized' as women often do not want to admit that they are depressed in case their babies are taken into care
- that the intervention is giving emotional support to women in terms of social as well as psychological need
- that 12 of the 13 health visitors questioned reported a high level of confidence in the use of non-directive counselling to manage PND
- the intervention has resource implications. The programme is demanding of scarce health visiting time and has to compete with the many other priorities health visitors have in their day-to-day practice. Weekly visits offering non-directive counselling continue well beyond eight weeks, the time when intensive home visits are usually diminishing
- that a support group was started in the locality; however, there were limited facilities with no crèche, transport problems and the scheme did not work out
- health visitors need to be sensitive to the women's literacy ability. Some of the women could not read the questionnaire and had to be helped to complete it.

Prior needs assessment   A survey carried out in early 1992 showed a high incidence of postnatal depression in areas of social disadvantage within the locality. A further survey carried out over a three-month period in the summer of 1993 analysed results from the Edinburgh Scale and found that postnatal depression in the locality was 13%. These findings are consistent with most studies in England and Scotland which have shown a remarkably consistent prevalence of 10–16%. Therefore the incidence in this area would appear to be within expected levels when shown as a locality average. However, closer scrutiny of the statistics revealed some very interesting findings. Results were produced by each health visitor's caseload.

Health Visitor X: incidence 25%
Health Visitor Y: incidence 30%
Health Visitor Z: incidence 7%

Caseload analysis of health visitors X and Y showed a high level of factors suggesting social and material disadvantage, whereas health visitor Z worked in a rural community showing very little indicators of social disadvantage and poverty. Given the magnitude of the problem particularly in areas of high social disadvantage together with the need to target resources to those in greatest need, there was a strong case for the proactive role which these local health visitors took in seeking out and offering support to those who suffer the misery of postnatal depression.

Characteristics of best practice in early detection and effective treatment of postnatal depression

- motivated, committed and skilled multidisciplinary staff
- practice based on a firm foundation of research and development
- use of standardized measurement of depression
- evidence of effectiveness and efficiency
- realistic aims and objectives
- use of effective quantitative methods
- multi-professional team working with shared goals and objectives
- empowerment of women fostering personal growth
- strengthening the capacity to cope
- improving the health and quality of life of the local women
- offering support and ways of coping for women with postnatal depression
- disseminating results
- monitoring and quality audit of health promotion
- developing partnerships and ways of joint funding with other agencies.

3   RESOURCES

Settings   Interventions are more effective when embedded in a variety of settings. For example, many successful interventions have involved home visiting with groups such as pregnant teenagers, breastfeeding mothers and lone parent families who are visited by health visitors, trained peers or lay health workers. Studies show that disadvantaged women with young children particularly valued the social contact provided by small group training sessions held at home. The importance of face-to-face interactions with individuals or small groups in an informal setting should also be promoted.

Importance of delivery agent   The people who are delivering the intervention are as important as the programme and its setting. Characteristics of the delivery agent should include skills such as leadership, knowledge of working with people, empowerment skills, motivation, organizational and communication skills, as well as vision, determination and stamina.

Training of delivery agents   Several interventions have been carried out by non-professional volunteers, often recruited from the target population and trained to offer support and guidance, or as peer education/support workers or to perform a task such as delivering a particular health message. Users and carers need training to promote access to reliable and accessible information to exercise their choice, independent training in advocacy to ensure confidence to put forward formal arguments, build effective leadership and competency skills and involvement in decision-making. Professionals can also be trained to provide smoking cessation techniques, for example, or emphasize the importance of training carers when they are running classes and programmes for older people or the disabled.

Use of support materials   Many of the programmes offer the use of educational materials such as booklets, CDs and videos. The impact of using such materials has rarely been assessed specifically. In some instances educational materials may be increasing inequalities in health and wellbeing. In many cases health education which aims to target individuals/communities encourages more involvement from higher social classes than those from lower social classes.

Example: Opportunity Youth

Settings   Opportunity Youth is an exciting innovative programme for 16- 18-year-olds who attend job skills training programmes within an inner city area. These young adults are generally from lower socio-economic groups and have a variation of abilities from the very limited to the exceptional. The majority are already habitual risk-takers in the areas of sexual activity, drug and substance abuse, petty crime, joy-riding and gambling. There is little to offer in the community for this age group, so they are reduced to life on the streets and are then prey to the influence of those of their peers who abuse alcohol, drugs and indulge in petty crime and joy-riding. Around 300 young trainees on job skills programmes access the workshops on a weekly basis and the programme aims to:

- promote personal development and health and social awareness amongst trainees in areas such as AIDS, HIV, and alcohol and drug use
- enable trainees to make informed and discriminating choices around health issues
- increase trainees' self-esteem and confidence
- enhance trainees' employment potential.

Importance of delivery agent   Peer education is the key to this programme which is about young people educating other young people. Peer educators assist in the development and delivery of the programme but most importantly develop relationships with the job skills trainees offering a befriending advocacy remit. Peer education programmes have been shown to enhance and help develop positive attitudes among young adults, and have proved to be an appropriate vehicle for health education, significantly more effective than a professional directed approach. The concept is simple and the impact can be much stronger than that using more traditional methods, especially with young people. Confidentiality is paramount in the relationships built between the project team members and the young people.

Training of delivery agents   The most obvious benefits of peer education are that, as young people themselves, they are more likely to gain credibility than professionals with this age group. Consequently, health messages are more likely to be listened to from an educator of the same age and social class who shares the same dress code, taste in music and social needs. The biggest benefit of all is using peer pressure in a positive way, which in itself is a powerful strategy for peer education and involves the sharing of information, attitudes or behaviours by young people who are not professional instructors but educators none the less. However, professional support and training is given from the health visitors and social workers. This allows the work that the peer educators initiate and the problems they identify to be developed by the professional team. Examples of problem areas have been worries about:

- Pregnancy and STD
- Homelessness
- Family problems
- Drug problems
- Threats of violence
- Disclosure of abuse.

The trainees' language demonstrates that they have assimilated the knowledge explored in group sessions and they have a high level of understanding of health, social and economic problems associated with smoking, alcohol, drugs, solvents, sexual activity and relationships. Trainees have a greater awareness of sources of information and support provided by the statutory and voluntary sectors in relation to health education.

Use of support materials   Opportunity Youth has become the most popular and most used source of information and advice in the areas of alcohol and drug abuse, solvent abuse and contraception for trainees. Trainees have produced a video on drugs based on their own experiences and knowledge gained in this area. It is intended for education use with other young people. Results of an evaluation suggest that there has been a significant drop in teenage pregnancies across the four workshops and over the last two years there has been a 66% reduction in incidence.

Characteristics of best practice in the Opportunity Youth programme

- decisions based on needs assessment
- multidisciplinary team
- identifying unmet needs in the young population
- research based project using peer education methodology
- involving local young people as trainees
- service provision sensitive to local needs of the young community
- viewing partnership with community agencies as a shared resource seeking to improve the social and health status of young person
- providing employment in the community
- providing a quality youth counselling service
- reducing inequalities in health and social care of the young
- playing an active role in improving the health and quality of life of the young person
- empowering the young
- sharing of information, attitudes and behaviour by young people
- offering support networks
- providing information in a user-friendly manner
- reducing teenage pregnancies in the area
- developing an innovative research methodology for assessing the health and social needs of the young people within the community
- strengthening the capacity of the young person to cope with peer pressures
- disseminating results and information sharing
- monitoring, report writing and evaluation.

---

4   INDIVIDUALS/COMMUNITIES

A holistic approach to health   This means viewing health and social need by looking at the 'whole' person or the community they live in. This contains many parts such as the physical, the spiritual, the emotional, the mental, the social and the environmental. Are you aware of the impact of unemployment, poverty and deprivation, poor housing, lack of education, inadequate nutrition, lack of social support and adequate ways of coping with life can have upon and individual's health and wellbeing? It is also necessary to look at the impact of rural health compared to urban health and the social network in which the individual lives such as those in the homeless community, those acting as carers, those living lonely isolated lives and the effects that these factors may be having upon their psychological and behavioural wellbeing.

Empowerment   This means providing effective health promotion that allows the individual or community to take control of their lives, their health and needs and to determine their own destinies, allowing them to take direct action in the process of change. Encouraging patients, clients and users to become involved in health development and decision-making means changing their attitude and that of professionals to allow active participation. Empowerment of individuals is visible in self-help groups where people can produce coping skills to reduce depression, allowing increased skills and personal contact and strengthening them to provide a better quality of life for themselves and their families. Empowerment can therefore be personal (increased self-esteem, increased coping ability) or collective, as in campaigning for better access to care and services on behalf of all.

Community development/commitment   Commitment to a holistic approach to health recognizes the central importance of social support and social networks. Individuals and communities need to be fully involved in partnerships and networks to set priorities, make decisions, plan strategies and implement them in order to achieve better health. An example of this is the Community Action Model which aims to mobilize disadvantaged groups to reduce the fact that inequalities and inequities may damage their health.

Culturally appropriate   Making sure that your intervention is sensitive to the cultural needs of the target group is vitally important with respect to communication and support.

Example: Lay Health Worker Project

A holistic approach to health   The Lay Health Worker Project was initiated in an area where traditionally food and housing had been very poor and there was a heavy dependence on public sector housing. Overcrowding was very much in evidence. There were high levels of truancy, juvenile delinquency, youth unemployment and teenage pregnancy in the area. The health experience of the local population paralleled the social and economic disadvantage of the area. It had a high infant mortality rate of 11.9 per 1000 births and the percentage of low birth-weight babies was 6.9% compared with an overall average of 5.8%. Lone parent families made up 25–30% of family units in the area. Health promotion and health education were clearly important in such a locality. However, the major problem was how to promote health in a way that was sensitive to and respectful of local people's values and circumstances. A holistic approach and one which recognized the wider social and environmental context in which health decisions were made was considered the best.

Empowerment   The main aim of the scheme was to promote health in the socially and economically deprived community by the empowerment and employment of local people. The intrinsic value of lay people's contribution to health was the most important feature of the scheme and brought with it many challenges and assumptions that were made from a service point of view, about 'clients', 'patients' or 'consumers of health'. From this it was hoped that:

- health would be improved in the community by the lay health worker who would provide an accessible source of health information not only in their paid work capacity but also by sharing information with family, friends and wider social networks
- the training of the lay health workers would build on their existing knowledge and experience, that their abilities would be valued and developed, leading to an increase in self-confidence and consequently an improvement in their employability
- funding would be secured for the long-term future of the project
- the public would feel more involved in the health service through its valuing of local people
- the lay health worker would become integrated into the community nursing service, without losing their lay perspective and professionals would see the value of lay opinion and develop community approaches in line with that view.

Community development/commitment   The project identified the real difficulties of empowerment and community development in practice, highlighting the tensions that may be aroused for professional staff. For some health visitors and district nurses, lay involvement in health promotion was not acceptable. Professional workers using the scheme reported being unsure about the aims of the project and the value of the practical support that it offered. The lay health workers brought the project a human face which was the key to its implementation. Families and individuals involved in the scheme valued the lay health workers and stressed the ease with which they could build relationships. Health promotion happened as the relationships developed. The project was about the relief of stress and anxiety, the building up of self-confidence and the improving of quality of life.

Culturally appropriate   The Lay Health Worker Project relied on innovation diffusion theory which stresses that the most powerful agents of change in any community are members of the local population who can act as sources of information on health and naturally relate to a wider social network of relatives and friends. The use of lay people in health is a major method of working in Third World countries as it attempts to bridge the gap between local health beliefs and customs and the newer 'western medicine'. There is normally inherent in the best projects a valuing of each other's position and joint learning about the appropriateness of the care offered. It is on this mutual respect that the Lay Health Worker Project was founded and attempted to develop in practice. It was always the intention of the project to develop a community-based role and it was this area that produced tremendous growth. The work was reaching all age groups in the community, e.g. mother and toddler groups, young women's groups, postnatal support groups, elderly people's groups, carers' groups, older women's groups, youth groups and travellers groups.

Characteristics of best practice in the Lay Health Worker Project

- working in partnerships between professionals and local communities
- involving local people
- empowering local people
- realistic aims
- overcoming resistance
- balance between the negative and positive factors involved in the project
- learning from experience
- training of lay staff and professionals
- playing an active role in improving the health and quality of life of the local community
- development of self-esteem and employment of lay health workers
- reducing anxiety and stress among carers
- disseminating results
- evaluation and monitoring.

STAGE 5:   WHICH MEASURES WILL BE USED?

Measurement

Measurement is itself evaluation because it is quantifying something by comparison with something else. Measures are often used in evaluation to quantify needs and outcome, but also to quantify inputs (e.g. costings) and processes (e.g. time, the number of defined visits). Measurement is an efficient way to communicate evidence and describe things. It is therefore essential in an evaluation that some form of measurement is used. The golden rule is to measure the objectives set up in the planning process. However, this can be more difficult when there is a multidisciplinary/multi-agency collaboration and increased involvement of the community. Such collaboration may require a more comprehensive set of criteria against which to evaluate progress.

Evaluation should be geared to the level of change most likely to occur as a result of the implementation of a particular programme (see case study, Chapter 13). Interventions should cover a diversity of topics areas and target groups. It is vital that all involved in the evaluation recognize that targets, planned measures and outcomes may change as the project progresses through time. The intention of most interventions is to bring about evidence of:

- health gains – knowledge, attitude and behaviour
- health impact assessments
- fair access

- effective healthcare
- efficiency
- a positive patient/carer experience
- positive subjective health gains
- health outcomes
- social changes in the wider environment or society
- empowerment of individuals or communities by improving their knowledge and skills in dealing with health and social need problems.

Always remember not to collect data which someone else has already collected. Check for secondary sources of collected data. There are different ways of searching for sources. The simplest way is to ask service providers, clerical staff or managers if there are records, statistics or other sources which might give the data needed for the evaluation. Also identify data already published in research reports and journals by searching databases such as MEDLINE, Bids, The Cochrane Databases, York Databases, Database of Economic Evaluations, Social Science Citations Indexes. Search methods are well described in Gray (1997). Remember also that national and local government collect data about populations, patient groups and public services.

When collecting data you must pay attention to the:

- clearly defined evaluation question/s
- theoretical basis of the measures
- clearly described setting of the evaluation
- interpretation of subjective meaning
- description of the social context
- attention to lay knowledge
- description of the sampling strategy and sampling methods
- scope of data collection and issues of subjectivity
- description of data collected
- consistency and reliability of the information collected
- tests for the validity of the results
- generalizability of measurement.

The above introduces us to terms such as sampling, consistency, validity and reliability. The reader with a research background will be familiar with these concepts and see them as part of the language used to describe features of data collecting methods. Those readers who find this terminology new to them should consult books and articles suggested in the further reading section. The most basic working definitions are given below.

Reliability is the extent to which a data gathering method will give the same results when repeated (consistency). For instance unstructured interviewing as a method can result in unreliable data.

Validity is the extent to which a measure or data reflects what it is supposed to measure or give information about. It includes terms such as internal and external validity as well as face, construct and content validity.

Both of these terms can be used in different ways and further reading about these concepts is recommended. For instance, qualitative methods can give more valid data than quantitative methods when investigating the subjective experience of health and wellbeing for individuals, but can be less reliable than quantitative methods. As we stated earlier, validity in qualitative process evaluation can be increased when using a triangulation method. Remember triangulation means collecting data from several different sources, perhaps using a multi-method approach, all of which work together to improve validity and provide an extended picture of the intervention with its successes and also its pitfalls. One method on its own may not be enough. Think of combining questionnaires and surveys, with structured interviews and focus groups (see case study in Chapter 10).

Sampling is another term often used in evaluation. It can be broken down into a wide range of types. Examples are given below.

Purposive/systematic sampling is when a sample of people are deliberately chosen.

Target sampling is when the targets of the intervention are identified.

Theoretical sampling is a specific technique for qualitative analysis and is based on grounded theory approaches.

Statistical sampling is used when an evaluation considers issues to do with representativeness.

We can never reach every member of a population but if we use smaller samples or target groups we need to know how representative this sample is of a larger population. Care needs to be taken in selecting a sample before gathering data for both 'internal validity' and in order to be able to make generalizations and valid inferences at a later date ('external validity'). The reader should consult books that describe the more sophisticated methods used for sample designs, such as 'random sampling,' 'quota sampling' and 'cluster sampling'.

Which measures will be used?

It is essential in any evaluation process to identify sources of data, obtain access to them and collect those data needed to judge the value of the evaluated. There is a range of methods which can be used for collecting data.

Observational methods: An unobstrusive observation of the participant and where appropriate of oneself. This is the main technique in many ethnographic and case study designs.

Interview methods: Interviews may be structured, semi-structured, or open and unguided. Data may also be collected using focus groups.

Survey/questionnaires: These may be small or large in focus and may use rating scales and more validated and standardized questionnaires.

Measurement methods: These should be holistic in nature and cover biopsychosocial and environmental issues. More subjective methods can be used in collecting data, and standardized instruments which have already been validated, such as disease-specific, wellbeing and quality of life measures, may be employed.

Data already collected: It is permissible to include data already collected within other interventions, by managers, other researchers, in audits, and other records and documents.

It is not within the range of this handbook to offer detailed instructions about how to use these methods. Stage 5 can only hope to provide a simple introduction to the various methods contained within the qualitative and quantitative methodologies. The further reading section refers the reader to general texts about research methods in health sciences, social sciences, nursing and medical research. Those wishing to extend their understanding of any particular method should consult more specialized texts. When referring to the methods, the handbook suggests various styles of collecting data and their relative strengths and weaknesses; however, the list is not intended to be inclusive or exhaustive, but rather should be seen as offering prompts to the evaluator. The handbook does not imply that some styles are more 'valid' than others or that there is a 'hierarchy of methods' or that some are 'hard' or 'soft'. Obviously, though, while looking at the strengths and weaknesses of the methods the reader should be able to assess that some are better suited to particular purposes, and that others will give more valid knowledge about specific issues.

Methods which can be used in collecting quantitative data and qualitative data are shown in Tables 8.2 and 8.3 respectively.

Having surveyed the various methods in the preceding pages it may be worthwhile now to consider some of the more practical points of data collection.

Practical points of data collection

Have you explored thoroughly the choice of methods?

There is generally no best method. The selection of methods should be driven by the evaluation question you are seeking to answer. This may be moderated by what is feasible in terms of time, resources, skills and expertise. What are the most important quality issues? Can you avoid bias? Is there relevant information elsewhere and can it be extrapolated to your intervention? Useful sources are local health promotion departments and local voluntary agencies.

What mix of methods (pluralistic evaluation) do you propose to use?

The virtues of multi-methods have been emphasized. As we point out, all methods have strengths and weaknesses and you are seeking to match the strength of one to the weakness of the other and vice versa. This may involve a degree of customization: for instance, the combination of an unstructured interview or focus group, with mini case studies linking to a questionnaire survey. Is triangulation possible? Remember the benefits are considerable: it is very useful for validity and reliability, it provides rich data and allows the user's voice or community voice to be heard.

Have you thought through potential problems in using the different methods?

What resources are available such as time, skills, equipment? How much experience has the intervention team in using the methods and understanding their strengths and weaknesses? Make sure that the setting you employ matches the styles of methods you are using. Do the methods raise any ethical issues? Pilot work may be necessary to bring out any problems.

Table 8.2 Methods which can be used to collect quantitative data

Features	Strengths	Weaknesses
Routine data collection Data collection at population level (Census, Government Surveys, National Surveys, ESRC Data Archive, Annual Reports, Evidence-based – Cochrane Centres, Systematic reviews) Useful for: Secondary Analysis Evidence-based information	Reliable valid as measures Available from other agencies reasonable complete Data on morbidity/mortality	Retrospective – most recent Census was 1991 Limited in scope May not include 'HARD TO FIND' groups such as women, elderly/retired minorities, those hospitalized, children
Collecting records from practice records Practice records and computer database Patient registers Audits of guidelines/protocols	Easy to retrieve Can identify groups with clearly definable characteristics	Timely, accuracy of recording Under-represents prevelance and is not fully representative of the practice population Completeness may vary e.g. functional dependency is often missing
Questionnaires Self-completion quantifiable scales Most common is Attitudinal Measurement Can be standardized or validated for specific purpose Useful for: Measurement of attitudes/knowledge/behaviour Assessment of need, health, illness, functional ability, psychological status and environmental issues	Very efficient in terms of evaluator time and effort Standardization = validity/reliability If constructed well, coding and analyses can be computer aided Randomization/sampling/controlling can be included	Limited check on honesty May lead to predetermined responses Interpretation may be problematic Requires factor analysis for validity/reliability
Randomized Control Trials (Gold Standard) The assignment of subjects to different conditions with manipulation of one or more variables (independent variables) and the measurement of the effects of this manipulation (dependent variables) while controlling all other variables. Useful for: Clinical setting, drug trials Evidence-based medicine	Provides evidence of causality Specifies randomization Uses comparison groups Valid/reliable Allows generalization of results Eliminates confounding variables	Double-blind procedures have to be used to reduce experimenter expectancy effects Not suitable for 'real world' Ethics of using a control group Must be well designed Expensive and problematic Artificiality
Quasi-Experimental Design An experimental design without randomization to experimental/control groups. Useful for: Comparing 'naturalistic' units such as schools/worksites	Allows 'Real World' research Allocates naturalistic units such as schools/worksites/communities to expt/control groups Does not require randomization Pre-and post intervention measures provides 'baseline' evidence	Lack of control because of lack of manipulation and randomization Causal relationships not included Can be expensive and time consuming

Table 8.3 Methods which can be used to collect qualitative data

Features	Strengths	Weaknesses
Postal survey Useful for: • Prevalence of ill health • Functional dependency • Socio-economic factors • Knowledge, attitudes • Use of and access to services • Linking all user groups • Advice about specific issues	Time required minimum No observer bias Quantifiable data if required Identifies difficult to find groups Reaches remote areas Identifies wide range of issues Pilot for survey Can cover embarrassing and sensitive issues	Variable return rate Costs involved in translation No explanation for issues Representativeness is known Selection bias: Young men tend not to respond Language barrier in some cases May exclude severely disabled both physically and mentally Damaging behaviours do not respond e.g. smoking, drug users

Focus groups
Useful for:
• Discussion groups of about
  5–15 people facilitated by a
  trained moderator and assisted
  by an observer
	Good exploratory work
	Good for testing theories
	Good for exploring 'why'
	people think in such a way
	Good backup to quantitative
	data
	Good for debate
		Time/costs may be high
		Criticised as subjective
		Training may be required
		Small numbers
		Lack of rapport with group
		Interviewer bias
		Not for use with:
		Those geographically dispersed
		Eliciting views from young or
		around personal/sensitive issues

Telephone interviews Useful for: • 'Hard to reach' groups	Speed of response quick Ability to target people living in geographical 'patches' Cost low	Training required to ensure all interviewers use same approach Interviewer bias
Observation **(Participant/Non-Participant)** Useful for: • Behavioural observation • Non-verbal cues • Interactional contexts • Team interaction	Can be systematic and objective Reduce sensitivity by several of the team doing the same thing 'Real life' data collection from naturalistic situation Directness – watch and listen Compliments other techniques Social response bias removed and memory deficiencies removed	Can be subjective/selective Record data immediately Observer bias effect Very time consuming Demands submersion into 'group'/community
Rapid Appraisal Useful for: Key informant interviews by observation, focus groups or interviews • Team approach • Assessment of needs of community • Project planning	Complimentary to qualitative issues Relatively quick 'In the field' Offers flexibility Examines health in socio- economic context Gives richness and user views Participants can set the agenda	Time, co-ordination Needs local practitioners to collect data – is this possible? Only scratches surface Very subjective/do not use alone Observer/selection bias Training requirements

Table 8.3 (Continued)

Features	Strengths	Weaknesses
• Social structure • Culture • Behaviours attitudes • Knowledge, perceptions • Defining problems • Feelings for key issues • Identifying resources/solutions • Identifying characteristics of area • Targeting groups/individuals	Consensus can occur Direct input of group	Requires input from multidisciplinary team and all other agencies to ensure action
Interviews May be structured, semi-structured or unstructured Useful for: • Assessment of need • Assessment of attitudes/ knowledge/behaviour • Defining problems • Identifying resources/solutions	Flexible and adaptable Provides rich and illuminating data Non-verbal cues help with understanding of the verbal response Allows follow-up of interesting responses Adjunct to quantitative	Time consuming Lack of standardization Concerns over reliability/bias Notes need to be written up immediately Cost / Time if using tapes (1 hour tape takes 10 hours Identifying and to transcribe)
Diaries A kind of self-administered questionnaire. Ranges from totally unstructured to specific questioning. Useful for: • Any area where direct observation or interviewing might be difficult or sensitive.	Minimum effort for getting substantial amounts of data May act as a proxy for observation Precursor to interviews	High responsibility on the respondent Prone to bias/subjectivity Needs same care as construction of a questionnaire Coding may be difficult
Case Studies Single case study involves 1 person Multiple case studies can involve a group/community/service, programme etc Useful for: • Focusing on contextual factors • Attitudes preceding an outcome • Exploring determinants, processes, experiences	Totally flexible Allows conceptual framework Exploratory theory building Naturalistic settings Holistic view of health	Seen as 'soft' technique Requires a sampling strategy Relies on trustworthiness of the evaluator
Ethnographic Study Study of a 'group' It seeks to provide a written description of the rules and traditions of a 'group/community'	Provides rich description Useful exploratory work to develop theories Real life evidence	Questions over reliability/validity Costly Timely Sampling difficult

Do the methods allow for the necessary flexibility and commitment?

In the early stages, you may wish to use methods which might need to be modified later in the evaluation, e.g. unstructured observation or interviews may move to more structured or standardized instruments at a later stage. Try to keep the possibility of a flexible approach in mind, and remember that a degree of commitment is important throughout. Data collection should be undertaken with the final understanding that results will need to be disseminated widely.

STAGE 6:   WHICH SUCCESS INDICATORS WILL BE USED?

It is beyond the range of this handbook to comment upon or define in depth every aspect of the 16 characteristics selected as indicators of a successful inequality intervention. However, the following Tables on page 125 provide some degree of organization of them and suggests cognate measures and methods of data collection. Those wishing to explore specific areas in detail should consult one or more of the following texts below. However, two of the most important measures for any evaluation is the assessment of 'holistic' health and 'community development'.

Measurement of 'holistic' health

Many concepts in evaluation such as health are difficult to operationalize. In many evaluations we use numerical data from measures to describe or explain. Numbers are an efficient way of describing processes, impacts and outcomes and allow us to see patterns and trends. For holistic health, measurement of outcomes can include:

- Physical functioning: activities of daily living, ability to walk, read, sleep, mobility scales, temperature, blood pressure, glucose levels etc.
- Psychological functioning: cognitive and coping abilities, self-esteem, depression, anxiety, helplessness etc.
- Social functioning: social support, networks, employment status, community participation etc.
- Environmental functioning: adequate housing and transport, access to leisure facilities etc.

It is not the intention of this handbook to describe these different measures in detail because they are well described in general texts such as Bowling's description of measuring disease (Bowling, 1995) and her review of quality of life measures (Bowling, 1991). Always check to see if a range of measures is available from elsewhere and after assessing their levels of reliability and validity look at their applicability for the purpose of your evaluation. This is important as it can save money, time, skills and can actually help you to produce more valid and reliable measures than you could construct yourself. Table 8.4 provides the reader with a number of scales and questionnaires which have been tested for validity and reliability and have been developed for a range of different types of health and biopsychosocial issues that may be the focus of a health promoting programme or intervention (see case study in Chapter 11).

However, health is a concept that means different things to different people and different professionals. If you decide to measure health outcomes as an appropriate component of your evaluation always make sure to select outcomes that are relevant to your objectives. This may seem obvious but it is very tempting to examine everything about a patient's/client's/user's health. There is a great advantage in selecting measures that have already been validated – the world does not need another 'quality of life' measure.

Subjective measures of health

Remember in many evaluations chronic illness and disability are not objectively measurable, so that reliance on objective measures (based on a negative definition of health) may fail to reflect fully the extent of the problem. In measuring both positive and negative health it is important to take the account of lay people's own subjective measures of their health (see case study in Chapter 10).

Positive measures of health

The vast majority of people in any population or community are not ill. Therefore, measuring only mortality and morbidity has certain drawbacks. Although it is difficult to measure positive health, care should be taken to include measures of mental illness with measures of mental health, and measures of health status with measures of social support and community involvement.

Measures of social support and social health are particularly important to midwives, nurses and GPs who see their contribution to positive health as an important aspect of their health promotion role. Table 8.4 illustrates a number of scales covering a more positive view of health and includes measures of:

- Functional ability
- Health status
- Health impacts
- Psychological wellbeing
- Life satisfaction
- Morale
- Coping ability
- Social networks
- Social support.

Examples of the above scales can be obtained from the holistic health measurement texts listed in Further Reading at the end of this chapter.

Table 8.4 Validated measures of holistic health for use in health promotion interventions

Measurement of functional ability
The Older Americans' Resources and Services Schedule (OARS)
 Multi-dimensional Functional Assessment Questionnaire
Activities of Daily Living Scales (ADL)
Advanced Activities of Daily Living (AADL)
Instrumental Activities of Daily Living (IADL)
The Stanford Arthritis Centre Health Assessment Questionnaire (HAQ)
The Arthritis Impact Measurement Scale (AIMS)
The Index of Activities of Daily Living (ADL)
Townsend's Disability Scale
The Karnofsky Performance Index
The Barthel Index (Physical functioning)
Rand Functional Status Index (Physical functioning)
The Quality of Wellbeing Scale (QWBS)
The Crichton Royal Behaviour Rating Scale (CRBRS)
The Clifton Assessment Procedures for the Elderly (CAPE)
Arthritis Impact Measurement Scale (AIMS)

Measures of psychological wellbeing
Zung's Self Rating Depression Scale
Montgomery-Asberg Depression Scale (MADRS)
Hamilton Depression Scale
The Beck Depression Inventory (BDI)
Hospital Anxiety and Depression Scale (HAD)
State/Trait Anxiety Scale
The Symptoms of Anxiety and Depression Scale (SAD)
Goldberg's General Health Questionnaire (GHQ)
The Geriatric Mental State (GMS)
Geriatric Depression Scale
Short Mental Confusion Scales
The Mental Status Questionnaire (MSQ)
The Abbreviated Mental test Score (AMT)
Health Locus of Control
Quality of Wellbeing Scale
Sense of Coherence Scale (Subjective Wellbeing/Quality of Life)

Measuring social networks and social support
Inventory of Social Supportive Behaviours (ISSB)
Arizona Social Support Interview Schedule (ASSIS)
Perceived Social Support from Family and Friends
Social Support Questionnaire
Interview Schedule of Social Interaction (ISSI)
The Social Network Scale (SNS)
The Family Relationship Index (FRI)
The Social Support Appraisals Scale (SS-A)
Social Support Behaviours Scale (SS-B)
Interpersonal Support Evaluation List (ISEL)
The Network Typology: the Network Assessment Instrument
Loneliness Scale – UCLA
Social Support Scale
Social Support Availability and Adequacy Scale
Social Adjustment Scale
Social Support in the Adjustment of Pregnant Adolescents

Table 8.4 (Continued)

Measures of life satisfaction and morale
The Life Satisfaction Index A and B
The Life Satisfaction Index Z – 13-item version
The Affect-Balance Scale (ABS)
The Philadelphia Geriatric Centre Morale Scale (PGCMS)
The General Wellbeing Schedule (GWBS)
Sense of Coherence Scale (SOC)
Scales of Self-Esteem
The Self-Esteem Scale

Broader measures of health status
The Sickness Impact Profile (SIP)
The Nottingham Health Profile (NHP)
The McMaster Health Index Questionnaire (MHIQ)
Patient Satisfaction
Caregiver Quality of Life Index (CQLI)
Physical Health Battery
Mental Health Battery
Depression Screener
Social Health Battery
Life Events Scale
Gay Life Events Scale
Ward Atmosphere Scale
Community-oriented Programmes Environment Scale
Group Environment Scale
Coping Health Inventory for Parents (CHIP)
General Health Perceptions Battery
General Health Questionnaire (GHQ)
Malaise Questionnaire
The Short Form-36 Health Survey Questionnaire (SF-36)
The Short Form-12 Health Survey Questionnaire (SF-12)
The Dartmouth COOP Function Charts
The Cornell Medical Index (CMI)
Spitzer's Quality of Life Index (QL)
Linear Analogue Self Assessment (LASA)
The McGill Pain Questionnaire (MPQ)

Adult Patterns of Tobacco Use
Tobacco and Alcohol Use among Secondary School Children

Measurement of community development

Community development is identified as a method supporting capacity for social change in communities. It usually involves an interaction between communities, the statutory and voluntary sector, to empower people to work collectively and collaboratively (see case study, Chapter 12). Community development supports community-led action on problems, which the community has identified, and the achievement of change in relation to these problems, which communities identify. It is based firmly on a 'holistic' view of health, encompassing social, physical, behavioural, economic, and environmental dimensions. The approach emphasizes that these dimensions are interrelated and that people individually or collectively have their health needs met when these are maintained in sustainable equilibrium.

Planners and evaluators should agree on what is meant by the term 'community'. The concept of community is not limited to geographical location such as town, county or district. Community may also refer to a selected sub-population such as racial, ethnic, gender, or religious groups or to a location such as clinical area, hospital ward, school or worksite. In an evaluation of community development programmes, it has been argued that intervention success cannot be adequately assessed by health measures taken from individuals in that community (Hawe, 1995). This would not adequately capture the nature of community development outcomes. Success is linked with changes in the community itself, its networks, its ownership of community issues, impacts upon health and social need, perceived and actual empowerment in health and social issues.

Systematic measurements are still in their infancy but some evaluators have developed measures of community strength, community competence, community commitment and community empowerment (Swift, 1987; Goeppinger, 1995). This is an exciting new area and these developments may encourage health workers to think about what they are trying to achieve as a longer-term ultimate goal.

FURTHER READING

Stage 4

Arblaster, L., Lambert, M., Entwhistle, M., Fullerton, D., Sheldon, T. and Watt, I. (1995) *Review of the Effectiveness of Health Service Interventions to Reduce Inequalities in Health*, CRD Report, no. 3. York NHS Centre for Reviews and Dissemination.

Balarajan, R. (1995) Ethnicity and variations in the nation's health. *Health Trends*, 27:114–119.

Barr, A., Hashagen, S. and Purcell, R. (1996) *Measuring Community Development in Northern Ireland: A Handbook for Practitioners*. Voluntary Activity Unit, DHSS (NI): The Stationery Office.

Barr, A., Hashagen, S. and Purcell, R. (1996) *Monitoring and Evaluation of Community Development in Northern Ireland: a Handbook for Practitioners*. Voluntary Activity Unit, DHSS (NI): The Stationery Office.

Benzeval, M. (1995) *Tackling Inequalities in health: An Agenda for Action*. London: The Kings Fund.

Bullen, N. (1996) Defining localities for health profiling a GIS approach. *Social Science and Medicine*, 309: 781–784.

Catford, J. (1993) Auditing health promotion: what are the vital signs of quality? *Health Promotion International*, 6(2): 67–68.

Dale, A. and Marsh, M. (1993) *The 1991 Census User's Guide*. London: HMSO.

Eng, E. (1992) Community empowerment: the critical base. *Family and Community Health*, 15: 1–12.

Gepkens, A. and Gunning-Schepers, L.J. (1995) *Interventions to Reduce Socio-economic Health Differences*. Amsterdam: Institute of Social Medicine, University of Amsterdam.

Goeppinger, J. (1995) Community competence: a positive approach to needs assessment. *American Journal of Community Psychology*, 13(5): 507–523.

Harris, A (1997) *Needs to Know: A Guide to Needs Assessment for Primary Care*. London: Churchill Livingstone.

Hawe, P. (1995) *Evaluating Health Promotion: A Healthy Worker's Guide*. Sydney: MacLennan.

Lazenbatt, A. (1997a) *THSN, Volume 1: The Contribution of Nurses, Midwives and Health Visitors*. DHSS, Northern Ireland: The Stationery Office.

Lazenbatt, A. (1997b) *The Contribution of Nurses, Midwives and Health Visitors – A Directory of Survey Respondents*. DHSS, Northern Ireland: The Stationery Office.

Lazenbatt, A. (2000) Tackling inequalities in health in Northern Ireland. *Community Practitioner*, 73(2): 481–483.

Lazenbatt, A. and Hunter, P. (2000) 'An evaluation of a drop-in centre for working women'. Queen's University of Belfast/Royal College of Nursing, Northern Ireland.

Lazenbatt, A. and Orr, J. (2001) Evaluation and effectiveness in practice. *International Journal of Nursing Practice*, 7(6) (in press).

Lazenbatt, A., McWhirter, L., Bradley, M. and Orr, J. (1999) The role of nursing partnership interventions in improving the health of disadvantaged women. *Journal of Advanced Nursing*, 30 (6): 1280–1288.

Lazenbatt, A., McWhirter, L., Bradley, M. and Orr, J. (2000a) Community nursing achievements in targeting health and social need. *Nursing Times Research*, 5(3): 178–192.

Lazenbatt, A., McWhirter, L., Bradley, M., Orr, J. and Chambers, M. (2000b) Tackling inequalities in health and social wellbeing – evidence of 'good practice' by nurses, midwives and health visitors. *International Journal of Nursing Practice*, 6(2), April: 76–88.

Lazenbatt, A., Sinclair, M., Salmon, S. and Calvert, J. (2001) Telemedicine as a support system to Encourage Breastfeeding in Northern Ireland: a case study design. *Journal of Telemedicine and Telecare* (in press).

Lazenbatt, A., Lynch, U. and O'Neill, E. (2001b) Revealing the hidden 'troubles' in Northern Ireland: the role of Participatory Rapid Appraisal. *Health Education Research* (in press).

Leventhal, M. (1993) *An Introductory Guide to the 1991 Census*. London: HMSO.

Macdonald, G. (1996) Where next for evaluation? *Health Promotion International*, 11: 34–48.

Nutbeam, D. (1996) Achieving 'best practice' in health promotion: improving the fit between research and practice. *Health Education Research*, 11(3): 317–326.

Stage 5: Quantitative methods

Abbott, P. and Sapsford, R. (1998) *Research Methods for Nurses and the Caring Professions*. Buckingham: Open University Press.
   A substantially revised edition dealing with the appreciation, evaluation and conduct of social research. Aimed at nurses, social workers, community workers and others in the caring professions, this text focuses on research which evaluates and contributes to professional practice.

Beech, J. and Harding, L. (1990) *Testing People: A practical Guide to Psychometrics*. Windsor: NFER-Nelson.

Birley, M.H. (1995) *The Health Impact of Development Projects*. London: HMSO.

Black, N. *et al.* (eds) (1998) *Health Services Research Methods*. London: BMJ Publishing.
   This is a multidisciplinary account of current knowledge about the key methods used to evaluate healthcare. It describes the uses and limitations of the principal methods. Each chapter makes suggestions for practical application.

Bowling, A. (1997) *Research Methods in Health*. Buckingham: Open University Press.
   This comprehensive guide to research methods in health describes the range of methods that can be used to study and evaluate health and healthcare.

Bryman, A. and Cramer, D. (1990) *Quantitative Data Analysis for Social Scientists*. London: Routledge.

Burns, N. and Grove, S. K. (1999) *Understanding Nursing Research*. Philadelphia, PA: Saunders.
   The second edition of this AJN Book of the Year introduces readers to each step in the nursing research process, and shows them how to read, summarize, critique, and use the findings in

clinical practice. The authors, both published nurse researchers, employ a consistent style and a nursing-oriented approach that features highlights from published research studies and critique questions to make this subject easy to understand, and enjoyable to read about.

Chambers, R. (1998) *Clinical Effectiveness made Easy – First Thoughts on Clinical Governance.* Oxford: Radcliffe Medical Press.

Clamp, C. G.L. and Gough, S. (1999) *Resources for Nursing Research.* London: Sage.
Fully revised and updated, the third edition of this invaluable bibliography of sources of literature for nurses, includes over 2,760 entries, 64% of which are new. This comprehensive yet concise guide is designed for convenience and ease of use and covers all aspects of nursing and allied health research with accessible and informative entries compiled within three sections. The first covers the process of literature searching, using libraries and tools – print and electronic. In the second methods of inquiry are presented. The final section discusses issues surrounding nursing research.

Clifford, C. (1997) *Nursing and Health Care Research.* London: Prentice Hall.
A guide to nursing and healthcare, this book aims to take more account of healthcare professionals outside nursing and pay more attention to qualitative research and increased consideration of how to develop reliability and validity in research tools.

Costings, C. and Springett, J. (1995) *A Conceptual Evaluation Framework for Health-related Policies in the Urban Context.* Liverpool: Institute for Health Liverpool, John Moores University.

Crombie, I. (1996) *The Pocket Guide to Critical Appraisal.* London: BMJ Publishing.

Gray, M. (1997) *Evidence-based Healthcare.* London: Churchill Livingstone.

Grebich, C. (1998) *Qualitative Research in Health.* London: Sage.
A practical introduction to the main theories and methods of qualitative research for the health sciences is offered in this book. It covers the full range of conventional and new qualitative methods including ethnography, phenomenology, grounded theory, biography, action research, historical research, discourse analysis and post-modern, poststructuralist and feminist approaches to research.

Greenhalgh, T. (1997) *How to Read a Paper. The Basis of Evidence-based Medicine.* London: BMJ Publishing.

Hoinville, G. (1977) *Survey Research Practice.* London: Heinemann.

McIntosh, J. (ed.) (1999) *Research Issues in Community Nursing.* London: Macmillan.
This work brings together examples of research into aspects of community care. The research is presented in such a way as to inform nurses about developments and initiatives nationwide at the same time as laying down exemplar for the evaluation of other new developments as and when they arise.]

Muir Gray, J.A. (1997) *Evidence-based Healthcare: How to Make Health Policy and Management Decisions.* Edinburgh: Churchill-Livingstone.

Mulrow, CD. (1994) *Cochrane Collaboration Handbook* (updated September 1997). Oxford: Update Software.

NHS Centre for Reviews and Dissemination (1996) *Undertaking Systematic Reviews of Research on Effectiveness.* CRD Report; 4. NHS Centre for Reviews and Dissemination, York.

Oppenheim, A.N. (1966) *Questionnaire Design and Attitude Measurement.* New York: Basic Books.

Parahoo, K. (1997) *Nursing Research.* London: Macmillan.
Nursing is now a research-based profession. This means that all students need to become acquainted with the principles, mechanics and terminology of nursing research, understand why research is important, and how it is relevant to a 'practical' discipline such as nursing', learn how to evaluate other people's research and make use of research findings in everyday practice.

Payne, S. L. (1951) *The Art of Asking Questions.* Princetown: Princetown University Press.

Pilcher, D. M. (1990) *Data Analyses for the Helping Professionals: A Practical Guide.* Newbury and London: Sage Publications.

Polit, D.F. and Hungler, B.P. (1996) *Essentials of Nursing Research*. Lippincott, Williams and Wilkins.

This introductory nursing research text assists consumers in evaluating research findings in terms of their scientific merit and potential utilization. The text compares naturalistic inquiries (qualitative studies) and traditional scientific research (quantitative studies) with regard to each aspect of study. Research examples, both fictitious and actual, provide the student with opportunities to critically read and analyse the strengths and weaknesses of the studies in relation to concepts presented in each chapter. Two full research reports included at the end of the text facilitate the development of critical reading skills. This fourth edition features a stronger balance of quantitative and qualitative research and increased coverage of research utilization content – the steps in a research utilization project are identified and an example is provided.

Robson, C. (1993) *Real World Research: A Resource for Social Scientists and Practitioners*, Oxford: Blackwell Press.

Robson, B., Bradford, M., Deas, I., Hall, E., Harrison, E. and Parkinson, M. (1994) *Assessing the Impact of Urban Policy*. London: HMSO.

Sackett, D., Richardson, W., Rosenberg, I. and Haynes, R. (1997) *Evidence-based Medicine – How to Practice and Teach EBM*. London: Churchill-Livingstone.

Scott Samuel, A., Birley, M.H. and Ardern, K. (1998) 'The Merseyside guidelines for health impact assessment'. Liverpool: Public Health Observatory, University of Liverpool.

Thompson, D. and Martin, C. (2000) *Design and Analysis of Clinical Nursing Research Studies*. London: Routledge.

This text on the design and analysis of clinical research studies explains the basis of experimental design and statistics in a way that is sensitive to the clinical context in which nurses work. It uses data from actual studies to illustrate how to: design the study; use and select data; present research findings; and use a computer for statistical analysis. The scope of the study designs and associated statistical techniques covered in the book allow both the beginning nurse researcher and the more seasoned nurse investigator to approach a research study with confidence and optimism. The authors show how qualitative data can be approached quantitatively, what the advantages of this are from the nursing viewpoint, and how quantitative methodology can help nurses to develop a common language with other disciplines involved in patient care.

Vanclay, F. and Bronstein, D.A. (1995) *Environmental and Social Impact Assessment*. Chichester: Wiley.

Young, A., *et al.* (2001) *Connections; Nursing Research, Theory and Practice*. St Louis, MO: Mosby Publishing Company.

This text discusses theory and research, the importance of the connection between the two, and the inter-linking cyclical connection between clinical practice, research and theory. Core chapters review major nursing theories, research tools related to each theory, review of research conducted to support or advance each theory, and ideas for continued research. Finally, the text includes select reliable and valid nursing theory research tools to be used for research. The text aims to be more than theory and research text; it offers students help in the research process to make the connection between a real-world clinical question, nursing theory, appropriate research tools, and actual research.

Stage 5: Qualitative methods

Burgess, R. G. (1984) *In the Field: An Introduction to Field Research*. London: Allen and Unwin.

Fetterman, D. (1989) *Ethnography Step-by-Step*. Newbury and London: Sage.

Maykut, P. and Morehouse, R. (1994) *Beginning Qualitative Research: A Philosophical and Practical Guide*. London: Falmer.

Miles, M.B. and Huberman, A.M. (1984) *Qualitative Data Analysis: A Source Book of New Methods*. Newbury Park and London: Sage.

Patton, M. Q. (1990) *Qualitative Evaluation Research Methods*. Newbury and London: Sage.

Pilcher, D. M. (1990) *Data Analyses for the Helping Professionals: A Practical Guide*. Newbury and London: Sage.

Pope, C. and Mays, N. (1995) Researching the parts other methods cannot reach: an introduction to qualitative methods in health and health service research. *British Medical Journal*, 311: 42–45 (first of six articles on qualitative methods).

Pope, C. and Mays, N. (1995) Rigor and qualitative research. *British Medical Journal*, 311: 109–112.

Pope, C. and Mays, N. (1995) Observational methods in health care settings. *BMJ* 311: 182–184.

Robson, C. (1993) *Real World Research: A Resource for Social Scientists and Practitioners*. Oxford: Blackwell.

Strauss, A. L. (1990) *Sources of Qualitative Research and Grounded Theory Techniques*. Newbury and London: Sage.

Tesch, R. (1990) *Qualitative Research – Analysis of Types and Software Tools*. London: Falmer.

Yin, R.K. (1989) *Case Study Research: Design and Methods*, 2nd edn. Newbury Park and London: Sage.

Stage 6: 'Holistic' health measurement texts

Bowling, A. (1991) *Measuring Health: A Review of Quality of Life Measurement Scales*. Buckingham: Open University Press.

Bowling, A. (1995) *Measuring Disease: A Review of Disease Specific Quality of Life Measurement Scales*. Buckingham: Open University Press.

Cleary, P.D. (1997) Subjective and objective measures of health: which is better when? *Journal of Health Services Research and Policy*, 2(1), 3–4.

Funnell, R. (1995) *Towards Healthier Alliances – A Tool for Planning, Evaluating and Developing*. London: Health Education Authority.

Goeppinger, J. (1995) Community competence: a positive approach to needs assessment. *American Journal of Community Psychology*, 13(5): 507–523.

Hawe, P. (1995) *Evaluating Health Promotion: A Healthy Workers Guide*. Sydney: MacLennan.

Hunt, S. (1985) Measuring health status: a new tool for clinicians and epidemiologists. *Journal of the Royal College of General Practitioners*, 35: 185–188.

Stewart, A.L., Ware, J.E. (eds) (1992) *Measuring Functioning and Wellbeing: The Medical Outcomes Study Approach*. London: Duke University Press.

Voluntary Activity Development Branch (1996) *Guidance on the Commissioning and Conduct of Evaluations of Voluntary Organizations by Northern Ireland Government Departments*. DHSS, Northern Ireland.

Voluntary Activity Unit (1996) *Monitoring and Evaluation of Community Development in Northern Ireland*. DHSS, Northern Ireland.

Ware, J. (1992) The MOS 36-item short form health survey (SF36). *Medical Care*, 30: 473–483.

Wilkin, D. (1992) *Measures of Need and Outcome for Primary Health Care*. Oxford: Oxford University Press.

Stage 6: Community development measurement texts

Connor, A. (1993) *Monitoring and Evaluation Made Easy – a Handbook for Voluntary Organizations*. London: HMSO.

Gilchrist, A. (1995) *Community Development and Networking*. London: Community Development Foundation.

Goeppinger, J. (1995) Community competence: a positive approach to needs assessment. *American Journal of Community Psychology*, 13(5): 507–523.

Hawe, P. (1995) *Evaluating Health Promotion: A Healthy Workers Guide*. Sydney: MacLennan.

Health Canada (1996) *Guide to Project Evaluation – A Participatory Approach*. Ontario, Canada.

Kennedy, A. (1997) *Evaluating Community Development for Healthy Cities*. Copenhagen: WHO/EURO.

Kennedy, A. (1997) *Evaluating Community Development for Healthy Cities – A Practitioner's Guide*. Geneva: WHO/EURO.

Maltrud, K., Polacsek, M. and Wallerstein, N. (1996) *A Workbook for Participatory Evaluation of Community Initiatives*. Mexico: University of New Mexico.

Parish, R. (1995) *Quality in Health Promotion*. Copenhagen: WHO.

Rootman, I. (1997) A Framework for Evaluation of Health Promotion Activities. Toronto: Centre for Health Promotion, University of Toronto.

Rootman, I. (1999) *Evaluating Health Promotion*. Copenhagen: WHO/EURO.

Springett, J. (1998) *Practical Guidance on Evaluating Health Promotion*. Copenhagen: WHO/EURO.

Voluntary Activity Branch (1996) *Guidance on the Commissioning and Conduct of Evaluations of Voluntary Organizations*. DHSS, Northern Ireland.

Voluntary Activity Branch (1996) *Monitoring and evaluation of community development*. DHSS, Northern Ireland.

Stage 6

Blaxter, M. (1995) *Consumer Issues within the NHS*. London: Department of Health.

Bowling, A. (1991) *Measuring Health: A Review of Quality of Life Measurement Scales*. Buckingham: Open University Press.

Bowling, A. (1991) *Measuring Disease: A Review of Disease-specific Quality of Life Measurement Scales*. Buckingham: Open University Press.

Bullen, N. (1996) Defining localities for health planning: a GIS approach. *Social Science and Medicine*, 309: 781–784.

Carr-Hill, R. (1987) The inequalities in health debate: a critical review of the issues. *Journal of Social Policy*, 16: 509–542.

Carstairs, V. (1989) Deprivation and mortality: an alternative to social class? *Community Medicine*, 11: 210–219.

Cleary, P.D. (1997) Subjective and objective measures of health: which is better when? *Journal of Health Services Research and Policy*, 2(1): 3–4.

Eng, E. (1992) Community empowerment: the critical base. *Family and Community Health*, 15: 1–12.

Goeppinger, J. (1995) Community competence: a positive approach to needs assessment. *American Journal of Community Psychology*, 13(5): 507–523.

Hawe, P. (1995) *Evaluating Health Promotion: A Healthy Workers Guide*. Sydney: MacLennan.

Hunt, S. (1985) Measuring health status: a new tool for clinicians and epidemiologists. *Journal of the Royal College of General Practitioners*, 35: 185–188.

Jarman, B. (1983) Identification of under-privileged areas. *British Medical Journal*, 286: 1705–1708.

Kari, N. (1991) The Lazarus project: the politics of empowerment. *The American Journal of Occupational Therapy*, 45: 223–224.

McIver, S. (1993) *Obtaining the views of Users of Primary and Community Health Care Services*. London: Kings Fund.

Stewart, A.L. and Ware, J.E. (eds) (1992) *Measuring Functioning and Wellbeing: The Medical Outcomes Study Approach*. London: Duke University Press.

Swift, C. (1987) Empowerment: an emerging mental health technology. *Journal of Primary Prevention*, 8(1): 71–94.

Townsend, P., Phillimore, P. and Beattie, A. (1988) *Health and Deprivation: Inequality and the North*. London: Croom Helm.

Voluntary Activity Development Branch (1996) *Guidance on the Commissioning and Conduct of Evaluations of Voluntary Organizations by Northern Ireland Government Departments*. DHSS (NI): The Stationery Office.

Ware, J. (1992) The MOS 36-item short form health survey (SF36). *Medical Care*, 30: 473–483.

Wilkin, D. (1992) *Measures of Need and Outcome for Primary Health Care*. Oxford: Oxford University Press.

APPENDIX

Success indicators

Success indicators	Measures	Data collection
Approaches/partnerships		
Health alliances/inter-agency	Commitment Community participation Communication Joint working Accountability	Observation, interviews, questionnaires, focus groups, community records, organizational records
Multidisciplinary	Support Commitment Communication Team building Education	Interviews, questionnaires, reports, records, focus groups, diaries, observation
Multifaceted	Stepped care Combined treatments	Interviews, questionnaires, observation, records, focus groups
Intensive approach	Vigorous/orchestrated	Questionnaires, records
Tools (methods)		
Audit	Standards Guidelines Objectives Peer review	Questionnaires, focus groups, records, interviews, practice records, postal survey, telephone interview
Evaluation	Effectiveness Efficiency Equity Economy	Systematic reviews, databases, questionnaires, interviews, focus groups, secondary data, patient records, diaries, postal survey
Research-based	Qualitative/quantitative Health impacts	RCTs, quasi-experimental, interviews, case study, focus groups
Needs assessment	Deprivation Epidemiological Health status Social/environmental	Rapid appraisal Practice records Questionnaires/surveys Focus groups/key informants

Success indicators	Measures	Data collection
Resources		
Settings	Informal	Observation, focus groups
	Face-to-face	Interviews
Delivery Agent	Competency skills	Questionnaires, observation
	Leadership	Rating scales, focus group
	Motivation	Semi-structured interviews
	Organizational skills	Case study, diaries
	Communication skills	
Training delivery agent	Training schemes	Records, focus groups
	Support/guidance	Peer interviewing
	Peer education	
Support materials	Educational/training	Practice records, community
	Booklets/videos	records, interviews,
		focus groups, questionnaires
Individual/community		
Holistic health	Clinical/epidemiological	Patient records/interviews
	Behavioural	Questionnaires, surveys
	Social	Standardized questionnaires
	Psychological	Ethnography
	Subjective	Focus groups, diaries,
		interviews, case studies
Community development	Community empowerment	Focus groups, questionnaires,
	Quality of life	Observation, existing records,
		Community group records
Empowerment	Individual empowerment	Focus groups, interviews, questionnaires
	Community empowerment	Observation, community records
Cultural needs	Barriers	Rapid appraisal, focus groups,
	Equity	Interviews, questionnaires,
	Needs	Ethnography

CHAPTER 9

WORKING THROUGH AN EVALUATION: OUTCOME

STAGE 7: WHAT DO THE MEASURES SHOW? RESULTS

Outcome measurement

The measurement of outcomes is probably the most challenging task in evaluation. Although difficult to measure, reductions or impacts upon inequalities in health and social need should be seen as the gold standard for success in an inequality intervention (see case study, Chapter 13). An evaluation that seeks to establish a link between an intervention and its outcomes is said to be a 'summative evaluation', purely because it sums up the effects of the change. You must remember that health outcomes in any intervention may not just be a result of that particular intervention but may also be attributed to wider social changes and policies.

Not all outcomes, however, can be summed up easily as they may result from a number of different avenues of information. They may refer to subjective responses from patients and clients, or judgments made by community workers and inter-agency organizations. However, altogether they should have a direct impact but combined relationship on people's health and social need (see Chapter 3, Health impact assessment). The outcomes of health promoting interventions should no longer be measured simply in terms of attitudinal or behavioural change. Outcome measures of holistic health should include subjective feelings of wellbeing and functioning relevant to the physical, psychological, social and economic life of the individual or the community as well the different stakeholders' perspectives of success.

There are several models and hierarchies which suggest how we should measure health outcomes (Tones *et al.*, 1993; King, 1996; Macdonald *et al.*, 1996). According to these models the results or outcomes of any evaluation should be perceived as immediate, intermediate or long-term outcome indicators of effectiveness, impact or quality and should assess the relationship between health promoting action and process and health outcomes. They are measured by means of:

- gains in holistic health and wellbeing
- gains in social wellbeing and functioning

- impacts upon or reductions in inequalities or unacceptable variations in health
- equity in the use of resources
- increased access to services for disadvantaged groups
- improved 'quality of life'
- reductions in 'risk-taking' behaviour
- improved patient/client satisfaction
- increased knowledge and skills
- attitudinal changes.

The most comprehensive overview of outcome evaluation is provided by Nutbeam (1998) who illustrates a framework for the definition and measurement of relevant outcomes to health promoting programmes.

The model shown in Table 9.1 identifies three different levels of outcome (immediate, intermediate and longer-term) which are the result of three broad types of health promoting action; namely, education, facilitation and advocacy. Within the model immediate health promotion outcomes comprise components such as:

(a) *Health literacy* improved health knowledge and motivation with respect to healthy lifestyles, greater knowledge and know-how about gaining access to health and other support services, increased skills and confidence to take part in everyday activities as well as political processes.
(b) *Social influence and action* improved community competencies and capacities as well as increased community participation in decision-making.
(c) *Healthy Public Policy and Organizational Practices* changes in health and social policies directed towards improved access to employment, services, benefits, housing and the creation of environments that are cohesive and supportive for health.

Table 9.1 A model of outcomes for health promotion action

Immediate		Intermediate	Longer-term
Health promotion action	Health promotion outcomes	Intermediate health outcomes	Health and social outcomes
1 Education	(a) Health literacy	(a) Healthy lifestyles	(a) Mortality Morbidity Disability
2 Facilitation	(b) Social influence and action	(b) Strengthened individuals/ communities/ alliances	(b) Functional independence Equity
3 Advocacy	(c) Healthy public policy and organizational practice/health impact assessment (HIA)	(c) Healthy environments/HIA	(c) Quality of life

Source: Adapted from Nutbeam (1998)

Examples of immediate outcomes for inequality evaluations

- A more developed understanding of the needs of customers, clients and patients and other interested stakeholders
- Consensus of views of partnerships and organizations with a common understanding about the dimensions of targeting health and social need
- The extent to which senior management is committed to combatting inequalities in health
- Changes that may have occurred in organizational and professional cultures – these would include changes in priorities between different values, shifts to a more holistic view of health
- The impact of inter-agency working and working within different disciplines within the health service and community.

The model suggests that at an intermediate level health outcomes can include components such as:

(a) *Healthy lifestyles* and personal behaviours which protect the individual from disease or injury or the risk of ill health (both physical and psychological)

(b) *Strengthening/individuals/communities and partnerships* by creating social cohesion and providing the infrastructure for individual and group social support

(c) *Healthy environments* and environmental factors which are created to facilitate access to services or reduce risks from hazards to physical safety as well as the establishment of better economic and social conditions that support social inclusion and decrease social exclusion.

Examples of intermediate outcomes Strengthening individuals within inequality evaluations

- Empowered staff and consumers who have the commitment and skills to contribute to the continuous improvement of and the reduction of inequalities in health
- Empowered user groups with increased knowledge/skills
- Positive changes in attitude for users
- Creation of social support systems and improved coping strategies for target groups
- Improved quality of life and self-esteem for target group
- Improved mental health with decreased stress
- Increased client/patient satisfaction
- Improved education, training and employment prospects

- Positive changes in health and social wellbeing status of patients and clients
- A user perception of the quality of information received and their general satisfaction with the development and implementation of the intervention
- Decreased 'risk-taking' behaviour.

Examples of intermediate outcomes
Strengthening communities within inequality evaluations

- Empowering communities
- Creating community regeneration/development
- Strengthening social networks
- Strengthening psychological health
- Improving local health promotion activities
- Improving access to services
- Improving up-take of screening and prevention services
- Improving local health information and support
- Effecting reductions in smoking behaviour
- Effecting reductions in accidents
- Decreasing teenage pregnancies and postnatal depression
- Improving mental health.

Examples of partnership outcomes
Strengthening alliances for evaluations

- Evidence of reductions in multidisciplinary barriers and more cooperative multidisciplinary working
- Genuine improvements in a range of targeted areas
- Improving information systems to provide both internal and external customers with the information they need to contribute to the planning, development, delivery and evaluation of an intervention
- Identifiable savings of wastage through getting it right the first time, more cost effective and equitable use of resources
- The capacity of all parties concerned to learn from good quality initiatives and the creation and use of networks for diffusion and learning.

Not all interventions will embark on longer-term outcome evaluation. Impacts and effects upon inequalities in health are likely to be gradual and probably will take time beyond that of the intervention. Immediate and intermediate outcomes by contrast allow effects to be demonstrated within a shorter timescale. Above are examples of:

- immediate impacts/effects (may be assessed as early as 6–9 months into the programme or intervention);
- intermediate impacts/effects which strive to strengthen individuals/communities and strengthen alliances (these can be assessed from 1 year into the programme or intervention).

Both the timescale and the examples of outcomes here are simply indicative. Variations within common sense limits are obviously possible. Such immediate and intermediate outcomes will clearly reinforce the indicators of 'best practice' and even before the intervention is complete should indicate that it is being conducted in an effective way.

Examples of longer-term outcome effects

It is important that the long-term goal of your intervention is to pursue both holistic health gains and equity. Many inequalities in health status can only be dealt with through wide societal and policy measures that will aim to reduce the social inequalities which in turn give rise to health inequalities. Longer-term outcomes are important even though they may occur several years after the intervention has been terminated. Health professionals can play an important role in bringing to the attention of purchasing authorities evidence of inequalities in health and social care and in highlighting those policies that should be working with deprived groups in society to improve their overall health and their access to effective healthcare provision. Nutbeam's (1998) model suggests that:

(a) Reductions in mortality and morbidity and levels of disability represent longer-term health impacts/outcomes
(b) Functional independence and equity is the bridge between health and social impacts/outcomes
(c) Quality of life covers the broader social impacts/outcomes.

This model provides a sound basis for the development of a broad range of indicators for the outcomes of health promoting action (Figure 9.1). However, at present there is insufficient evidence to support the causal links proposed between these three levels. We need to build the knowledge base which concerns the links between the elements shown in Figure 9.1.

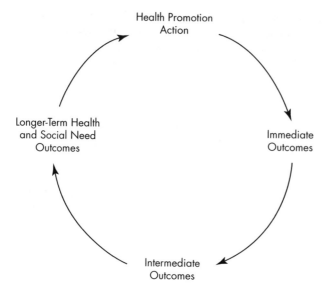

Figure 9.1   Health promotion

Longer-term outcomes: strengthening individuals

- Individual empowerment
- Empowered user groups
- Increased knowledge/skills
- Positive changes in attitudes and behaviour
- Creation of social support systems
- Improved coping strategies
- Improved education/training
- Improved self-esteem

- Improved quality of life
- Providing employment
- Decreased stress
- Decreased 'risk-taking' behaviour
- Improved mental health
- Reduced discrimination
- Reduced inequities
- Reduced inequalities.

Longer-term outcomes: strengthening communities

- Empowering communities
- Creating community development/ regeneration
- Strengthening social networks
- Strengthening psychological health
- Improving local health promotion initiatives
- Improving access to services

- Improving local health information/support
- Improving breastfeeding rates
- Improving child accident prevention
- Decreased mental ill health
- Effecting reductions in smoking

- Improving up-take of screening and prevention services
- Environmental change

- Reducing barriers and discrimination.

Longer-term outcomes: policy changes

- Major impact on health and environmental inequalities/inequities
- Improved access to services
- Anti-poverty lobby
- Welfare rights
- Road safety
- Smoking campaign
- Recognition of neglected population groups

- Environmental health
- Equal opportunities
- Employment opportunities
- Improvements in education
- Improvements in training
- Healthy eating
- Fair employment
- Crime prevention.

STAGE 8:   WHO SHOULD BE TOLD? DISSEMINATION

Dissemination network: sharing information

Having spent time and energy conducting an evaluation, it is important to ensure that the results and outcomes are disseminated as widely as possible. Sharing your work with others enables them to learn from your experience and apply the knowledge you have gained to their own practice. Evaluations are conducted for a variety of reasons, but mainly to provide information for decision-making and further funding. Chelimsky (1997) suggests that there are three main purposes for conducting evaluation, namely:

Knowledge-building   to cover the related questions which are generated by the evaluators to develop a sound explanation and better understanding of a specific area of health or social need.

Accountability   to provide evidence to improve performance and capacity and allow services and programmes to be strengthened.

Development   to provide a feedback component and allow the results of an evaluation to influence the on-going development of a service or a programme.

Reports and feedback mechanisms should not just be provided for funders and managers or for purposes of academic study but rather their content, language, and availability should reach all interested stakeholders or groups and should be disseminated as widely as possible. It is now widely recognized that 'getting research into practice' presents a major challenge. To be effective, however, you may need to report different kinds of information to different individuals or groups in different forms and at different stages of the evaluation. Remember that all reports should present problem areas and setbacks to provide future interventions with information about these obstacles. Think about how you should present your report, who should receive it and when.

What groups of people should receive information about the evaluation? These groups could be funders, managers, colleagues, users, teams, health authorities, universities, voluntary agencies etc. The information must be communicated to the appropriate potential users.

Should specific reports be directed at specific groups? Examples of such groups are user groups, patients, children, people with learning disabilities/mental illness, homeless people, travellers, lone parents, primary care professionals etc. Reports must address issues that the users perceive to be important and in a form that is clearly understood by the intended users.

When is the evaluation report required? Ensure that this is assessed at the beginning especially if required as part of a funding contract. Reports must be delivered in time to be useful for decision-makers.

Will there be interim report/s or should all information be released at once? Think of the costs (time, resources, expertise) involved at the outset.

Will the report be disseminated widely? Assess the costs – could the report be disseminated by newsletter, workshops, seminars, focus groups etc?

It is desirable to build a network of evaluation research in the area of inequalities to form an alliance of researchers, funders, health promoters, health alliances, health care professionals and most importantly representatives of those 'evaluated'. The evaluation team might consider a range of dissemination procedures such as academic publications, pamphlets, newsletters, peer networking, making presentations to different groups, arranging seminars, distributing summary bulletins, inequality working groups, community groups, voluntary mailing lists etc. It is important that the evaluation outcomes are visible as is active targeting of audiences with appropriately tailored information.

A database format for systematically collecting information about health promoting and health educating inequality interventions should be developed. The main areas to highlight should be: information about effectiveness of health promotion and health education activities; information on impacts and reductions of inequalities/ inequities in health and social need; and information about how these effects have been achieved as well as recommendations for improvements of health promotional activities. Think about engaging with others working on a similar inequality intervention to meet regularly, exchange progress reports and discover mutual benefits. You can also make presentations or send newsletters or summary bulletins to others to allow them to benefit from your work and avoid unnecessary duplication. At a local level, you can provide hospitals, community groups and libraries with your work to share information locally.

Understanding your primary audiences and users

Dissemination means more than just distributing a report. It involves the identification of key audiences, e.g. patients, clients, users, carers, other health practitioners, managers and organizations all working together to promote health. Before you embark upon a final report find out what the decision-makers consider are acceptable criteria for success. These may or may not correspond with your criteria for success. Also aim to find out in users' terms on what level they think the programme is expected to succeed. For a variety of reasons this all sounds easier than it is in practice.

For example, different users may want different information – even to answer the same question. A funding agency may require evidence from more reliable test data to prove that an intervention is succeeding, while those participating in the programme may wish for more anecdotal reports and responses from interviews. Other audiences may require both.

Some users expect the evaluation to support a specific point of view. Usually this is in the form of a user group having already made up their minds about the strengths and weaknesses of an intervention and they expect that the evaluation will only confirm their opinions. In reality the results of the evaluation may not support their preconceptions. Always alert users to your findings as they emerge, rather than in a final report to avoid the evaluator losing credibility. In fact, an effective evaluation report should contain no surprises.

For some users the information needs change during the course of the evaluation. It is not at all uncommon when a formative evaluation is well under way for the user group to identify some new information they would like to have. Although you cannot constantly alter your evaluation, consider reserving small amounts of resources to meet the requirements of the unexpected.

STAGE 9:   WHY REVIEW THE EVALUATION?

What are the strengths and weaknesses?

Assessing one's work is an important aspect of being a reflective practitioner. However, new or pilot interventions need a more thorough style of evaluation which includes negative findings (e.g. that a service, clinic was not appropriate; that community groups felt ignored and isolated) as well as positive ones (e.g. increased consumer/patient satisfaction, reductions in road traffic accidents). It is helpful to illustrate problem areas and barriers since doing so saves others from duplicating the same. Without evidence of efficiency, effectiveness, and equity it is difficult to argue that any intervention should become an established work practice.

It is important that all stakeholders are involved in reviewing the evaluation. All involved should question whether the chosen measures were right, the ease or difficulty with which the data was collected and, most importantly, whether the information gathered shed light on the questions all parties had about the intervention. In other words, did the programme meet its objectives, was it successful in reaching targets, did it impact upon inequalities in health and social need, did it improve equity and access to services and are changes to practice required? Health professionals have to accept the need to make changes to practice and service delivery.

Nurses, midwives and health visitors have an important role in helping colleagues to accept change. However, they need to be willing to accept new ways of working and let go of ways that are not effective. Kitson (1997) suggests that the key factors in changing clinical practice and community care are the involvement of practitioners, the management of the change process, the environment in which they take place, and the availability of a skilled change agent.

Recommendations should be clearly derived from the data, and spelt out to include difficulties, problem areas, barriers to implementation and lessons to be learnt. They should also be practical and capable of implementation.

You must also make sure that the conclusions have been tentatively rather than firmly drawn, as in many cases these are the only part of the evaluation report which people read. Rather than suggest a single remedy for weaknesses in the intervention, you might prefer to provide the users with options for alternative courses of action. Recommendations are not a wish list and should therefore follow logical judgments based on valid, reliable and objective data. This, after all is what evaluation is all about. Evaluation can help nurses, midwives, GPs, and other health professionals to:

- use evidence of 'best practice' as a basis for measuring their practice and care
- become involved in multi-professional evaluations as doctors, therapists and others must come to appreciate that effective processes of care and patient outcomes depend on good nursing care
- become involved in systematically examining the effectiveness of nursing practice
- become involved in inter-agency evaluations and partnerships with voluntary organizations
- accept the need to examine and change practice based on available evidence
- raise the profile of the user and client perspective
- highlight a more 'holistic' view of healthcare and produce sound evidence of how nursing can provide benefits to all stakeholders
- share with others knowledge and experience gained through the implementation of effective best practice.

FURTHER READING

Stage 7

Baker, M. and Kirk, S. (1996) *Research and Development for the NHS: Evidence, Evaluation and Effectiveness.* Oxford: Ratcliffe Medical Press.

Bowling, A. (1991) *Measuring Health: A Review of Quality of Life Measurement Scales.* Buckingham: Open University Press.

Bowling, A. (1995) *Measuring Disease: A Review of Disease-specific Quality of Life Measurement Scales.* Buckingham: Open University Press.

Bowling, A. (1997) *Research Methods in Health.* Buckingham: Open University Press. This comprehensive guide to research methods in health describes the range of methods that can be used to study and evaluate health and healthcare.

Bury, T. and Mead, J. (1998) *Evidence-based Healthcare: A practical Guide for Therapists.* London: Butterworth-Heinemann.

Chalmers, I. and Altman, D.G. (1995) *Systematic Reviews.* London: BMJ Publishing Group.

Cleary, P.D. (1997) Subjective and objective measures of health: which is better when? *Journal of Health Service Research*, 2(1): 3–4.

Crump, B.J. and Drummond, M.F. (1993) *Evaluating Clinical Evidence: A Handbook for Managers.* Harlow: Longman.

Dixon, R. and Munro, J. (1997) *Evidence-based Medicine: A Practical Workbook for Clinical Problem-solving*. London: Butterworth-Heinemann.

Entwistle, V., Watt, I.S. and Herring, J. (1996) *Information about Healthcare Effectiveness: An Introduction for Consumer Health Information Providers*. London: King's Fund.

Greenhalgh, T. (1997) *How to Read a Paper*. London: BMJ Publishing Group.

Jadad, A. (1997) *Randomised Control Trials: A User's Guide*. London: BMJ Publishing Group.

Hawe, P. (1990) *Evaluating Health Promotion: A Health Workers Guide*. Sydney: McLennan and Petty.

Jones, R. and Kinmouth, A.L. (1995) *Critical Reading for Primary Care*. Oxford: Oxford University Press.

King, J., Morris, J.N. and Fitz-Gibbon, C. (1988) *How to Assess Programme Implementation*. Newbury Park: Sage.

Lazenbatt, A. (2000) Tackling inequalities in health in Northern Ireland. *Community Practitioner*, 73(2): 481–483.

Lazenbatt, A. and Hunter, P. (2000) 'An evaluation of a drop-in centre for working women'. Queen's University of Belfast/Royal College of Nursing, Northern Ireland.

Lazenbatt, A. and Orr, J. (2001) Evaluation and effectiveness in practice. *International Journal of Nursing Practice* 7(6) (in press).

Lazenbatt, A., McWhirter, L., Bradley, M. and Orr, J. (1999) The role of nursing partnership interventions in improving the health of disadvantaged women. *Journal of Advanced Nursing*, 30(6): 1280–1288.

Lazenbatt, A., McWhirter, L., Bradley, M. and Orr, J. (2000a) Community nursing achievements in targeting health and social need. *Nursing Times Research*, 5(3): 178–192.

Lazenbatt, A., McWhirter, L., Bradley, M., Orr, J. and Chambers, M. (2000b) Tackling inequalities in health and social wellbeing – evidence of 'good practice' by nurses, midwives and health visitors. *International Journal of Nursing Practice*, 6(2) April: 76–88.

Lazenbatt, A., Sinclair, M., Salmon, S. and Calvert, J. (2001a) Telemedicine as a support system to encourage breastfeeding in Northern Ireland: a case study design. *Journal of Telemedicine and Telecare* (in press).

Lazenbatt, A., Lynch, U. and O'Neill, E. (2001b) Revealing the 'hidden 'troubles' in Northern Ireland: the role of Participatory Rapid Appraisal. *Health Education Research* (in press).

Macdonald, G., Veen, C. and Tones, K. (1996) Evidence of success in health promotion. *Health Education Research*, 11(3): 367–76.

Nutbeam, D. (1998) Evaluating health promotion. *Health Promotion International*, 13(1), 27–44.

Peckham, M. and Smith, R. (1996) *Scientific Basis of Health Services*. London: BMJ Publishing Group.

Sackett, D.L. (1991) *Clinical Epidemiology: A Basic Science for Clinical Medicine*, second edn. Boston: Little Brown and Company.

Sackett, D.L. (1996) *Evidence-based Medicine: How to Practice and Teach EBM*. London: Churchill Livingstone.

Stewart, A.L. (1992) *Measuring Functioning and Wellbeing – The Medical Outcomes Study Approach*. Durham and London: Duke University Press.

Tones, K., Tilford, S. and Robinson, Y. (1994) *Health Education: Effectiveness and Efficiency*. London: Chapman and Hall.

Stage 8

Burnard, P. (1992) Writing for publication: part of your career development. *Professional Nurse*, 7(12): 788–790.

Chelimsky, E. (1997) Producing credible evaluations of federal health programs. *Evaluation and the Health Professions*, 19(3): 264–279.
Hall, G.M. (1994) *How to Write a Paper*. London: BMJ Publishing.

Stage 9

Dunning, M. (1997) *Turning Evidence into Everyday Practice*. London: Kings Fund.
King, J., Morris, L. and Fitz-Gibbon, C. (1988) *How to Assess Programme Implementation*. Newbury Park: Sage.
Kitson, A. (1997) Developing excellence in nursing practice and care. *Nursing Standard*, 12(2): 33–37.
Leigh, A. (1991) *Effective Change: Twenty Ways to Make it Happen*. London: Institute of Personnel Management.
Wright, S.G. (1998) *Changing Nursing Practice*. London: Arnold.

PART THREE

CHAPTERS 10–13

EVALUATION TECHNIQUES IN 'PRACTICE' SETTINGS

It is now widely recognized that an understanding of evaluation methodology is essential for healthcare and nursing professionals. Nurses, midwives and health visitors as well as GPs must be able to evaluate their own practice and the practice of others. Not all practitioners will become researchers, but they should be able to appreciate the evaluation methods of others and understand how to incorporate evaluation findings into their own practice. The evaluation manual illustrates how evaluation is really an extension of what everyone does in everyday life when they want to know the answers to questions. To do this they ask questions, evaluate the information they are given before they decide to make use of it. Smith (1995) defines what signifies good evaluation as 'the judicious use of methodological imagination'. This means that it is not good enough to 'collect' data, that an evaluator must think long and hard about the nature of the intervention and the part that evaluation plays in shaping and interpreting it, what this means to consumers and patients and what is required to improve it.

The final section of this handbook in Chapters 10–13 contains a collection of examples of evaluation techniques, all concerned in some way with nursing or the study of health and community care. Evidence-based practice is now seen as central to the development of nursing as a profession. Each example covers the various stages of evaluation described within this manual, namely:

- Needs assessment (baseline measures);
- Structure;
- Process; and
- Outcome.

The examples are intended to illustrate the kinds of evaluation that can be undertaken by a small-scale evaluation team or a single practitioner with limited resources and all investigate various aspects of practice in the clinical field, within the community and in the voluntary sector. The four approaches show a diversity of qualitative and quantitative methods and each reflects the experience of applied evaluation as it occurs in practice, as opposed to how it looks in textbooks.

NEEDS ASSESSMENT
1. *Women's Health Needs Assessment Using Rapid Participatory Appraisal Techniques (page 141).*

STRUCTURE

PROCESS

OUTCOME

CHAPTER 10

EVALUATION IN PRACTICE: NEEDS ASSESSMENT

The following project provides a valuable case study to illustrate needs assessment or the collection of baseline information. Needs assessment is a practical research culminating in a description of a specific group or community's health and social need status, as well as the adequacy of resources available to that population. The process enables practitioners to uncover an unmet need or an under-served group within a community and use that information to design a solution to the identified problem. Rapid Participatory Appraisal (RPA) is a research process which deals with needs-based community assessments. It is a tool for participatory diagnosis and planning, culminating in the formulation of action plans with managers who have the resources to meet the identified need.

WOMEN'S HEALTH NEEDS ASSESSMENT USING RAPID PARTICIPATORY APPRAISAL TECHNIQUES

Background

The World Health Organization's (1978) philosophy of primary health care emphasizes the principles of community participation as enabling equity of provision based on intersectoral collaboration between communities and other services (e.g. health, social services, housing, environment). A public health approach to primary care involves working in partnership with communities to define their needs and shape services to meet those needs. The equitable provision of healthcare must begin with a systematic assessment of the needs of target groups and the setting of priorities in order to provide resources in the most efficient way to meet their respective needs. However, available resources are not always allocated equitably to assist different social groups who may be facing limited access and barriers to healthcare perhaps of a geographical, cultural, religious, and financial nature.

Working in partnership

The challenge for improving public health goes far beyond the dissemination of information about healthy lifestyles, preventative care, or even quality of care. At its roots, the challenge for public health calls for consumers to participate as full partners in the healthcare system, actively responsible for their own health maintenance and vigilant in demanding quality and cost-effectiveness (see Chapter 7, Stage 2). The principles of a community approach to any specific problem involve the participation in and ownership of agendas by all involved. This is obviously a departure from traditional methods of health assessment which use a more directive, top-down approach: experts define the problem, and then suggest solutions. The following description of the needs assessment in a disadvantaged area is based on the principle that people are experts on viewing their own environments, and this applies within the local context as much as anywhere else. Although examples of participatory research are more prevalent in developing countries (Scrimshaw and Hutardo, 1988; Thies and Grady, 1991; Ong, 1991; Shamian and Kupe, 1993; Varkevissor, 1993), this may be due to the misguided belief that poverty and ill health do not exist on the same scale in the developed countries of the Western world. Nevertheless, there would appear to be a need to apply the same techniques within locally defined areas. Moreover, it should be noted that, in spite of the rhetoric about public participation, a recent study (Poulton, 1996) found a marked unwillingness among some professionals to involve users in defining and planning services.

Needs assessment or baseline information

All evaluations require some form of baseline information or needs assessment measures to allow achievement to be measured against a yardstick or to act as a 'benchmark' (see Chapter 7, Stage 3). Community needs assessment activities should be carried out by health professionals, user groups and voluntary or community groups as a means of investigating the unmet needs of that community. Community may be defined as a geographical area where a group of people live and work. Communities can also comprise patient groups, clinic patients, school catchments, health authorities, people with shared interests and shared characteristics, such as those with disabilities (physical, learning and psychological), lone mothers, women, children, ethnic minorities, elderly people and those who are homeless or travellers etc.

In all evaluations there will be many different definitions of need and in some respects need is a subjective concept relative to a particular time and place. However, Doyal and Gough (1992) believe that individuals have objective needs, which are common to everyone. The strength of their approach is that it suggests a particular type of methodological framework for the kinds of auditing and profiling exercises which are currently carried out by many groups, particularly nurses. Doyal and Gough, like many nurses, believe that human needs cannot be argued away and that the first step in meeting needs requires a needs assessment which will draw on both top-down and bottom-up sources of information.

Doyal and Gough (1992) suggest 11 needs for all individuals:

- Adequate nutritional food and water
- Adequate protective housing
- Non-hazardous work environment
- Non-hazardous physical environment
- Appropriate healthcare
- Security in childhood
- Significant relationships
- Physical security
- Economic security
- Safe birth control and child-bearing
- Basic education

A variety of research instruments can be applied, from both qualitative and quantitative perspectives, in order to gain a multifaceted view of local needs (see Taylor and Bogdan, 1984; Patton, 1990; Bowling, 1997). Importantly, the main emphasis should be on the development of a method which is capable of involving the community in diagnosing needs and formulating an action plan. Always think about why you want to undertake a needs assessment.

Reasons for undertaking a needs assessment are to:

- provide baseline information for evaluation purposes
- provide decision- and policy-makers with justification for new programmes or services
- provide a rationale for reallocation of resources or budget priorities
- avoid duplication of efforts
- fill gaps in service delivery
- establish credibility
- establish 'good will' with target populations
- allow a proactive approach.

Limitations of official statistics

Most information available about the health of populations is published in official statistics and ranges from the entire nation to electoral wards. The ten-yearly (decennial) Census is a major source of baseline information on numerous population variables down to the smallest aggregate unit of approximately 200 households, known as an enumeration district. For further information see *An Introductory Guide to the 1991 Census* (Leventhal, 1993) and *The 1991 Census User's Guide* (Dale and Marsh, 1993). However, the most pertinent difficulty is that the Census is usually conducted every ten years and some urban areas, particularly those of interest to needs assessment studies, may change rapidly within one or two years. The Census is, however, invaluable in monitoring trends and showing where change has occurred.

Women are often underrepresented in official statistics (Blaxter, 1990; Lazenbatt *et al.*, 1999) which, although they provide wide coverage of the population, present only limited information regarding the socio-economic influences on the health of women and children. For example, little is known about the occupational influences on women's mortality because only a minority of female death registrations give details of the woman's occupation (Pugh and Moser, 1990). Within national surveys, women cannot be analysed as a single group in terms of class, because a significant proportion of those of working age do not have an occupation. As high a proportion as 36% of women of working age could not be allocated to an occupational class of their own from the information reported in the 1991 Census (Blaxter, 1990).

Why women's health?

Gender is an important determinant of health, as can be seen in health outcomes between women and men. Women have particular health needs because of their complex reproductive system and a need for fertility advice and control, pregnancy care and gynaecological treatment. However, in addition to biological factors, women's health is also affected both negatively and positively by social factors. Such factors include:

- responsibility for many roles to the extent that women's work has often been described as a 'double shift', with caring responsibilities in the family as well as outside work
- isolation
- fewer opportunities for education, employment and decision-making
- low pay and lack of independent income
- domestic and sexual violence.

This form of structural powerlessness can affect every aspect of women's lives, particularly education, employment, health promotion, housing and politics. There is now evidence to suggest that improving the health of women may help to improve the health of the community as a whole (Graham, 1993; Lazenbatt et al., 1999).

Poverty is also linked in several ways with behaviours associated with poor health. These 'unhealthy lifestyle' behaviours include smoking, over-eating, reliance on anti-depressants and tranquillizers as well as alcohol abuse. For example, studies of women and smoking suggest that unemployment and lack of opportunity are among the reasons why smoking is now so highly associated with poverty (Graham, 1988; 1993). Research suggests that factors such as cohesive social networks, community participation and self-esteem are closely related to improved health and psychological wellbeing and may be protective against the effects of stress (Cohen and Syme, 1985; Caplan, 1993; Wilkinson, 1996). It can be argued that in an unequal society it is the inability to participate that leads to damaged health and reduced quality of life (Save the Children, 1994).

Needs assessment using Rapid Participatory Appraisal Techniques (RPA)

One of the key issues within an evaluation process is how resources should be distributed, to reflect local needs. Traditionally, health services plan distribution on the basis of service use, but if needs are considered to incorporate felt, but not unmet needs, this approach may fall short. Accountability to local communities can become a reality as management and planning processes become more visible. Health within the area of inequalities in health is based on a total holistic concept to include an understanding of the person's physical, mental, social, and environmental wellbeing (see Chapter 8, Stage 6). This composite view moves far beyond the traditional medical definition. Factors which can contribute to a definition of holistic health should include:

Genetic make-up   Genes help to determine whether we develop disorders such as cystic fibrosis or spina bifida and our susceptibility to acute infections and chronic disorders such as heart disease and cancer

Lifestyle   The ways in which we treat our bodies (smoking, eating, drinking and exercising habits) are all powerful influences on our health, in the short and long term

Environment   The ecological, social, cultural and economic environments in which we live are both important direct influences on our health and powerful influences on the lifestyles we adopt

Access to services   Health services, screening and immunization services that prevent illness, treatment and care services that reduce the effects of illness and clearly influence our health, as well as other services provided by local authorities and voluntary organizations.

In order to tackle inequalities efficiently, individuals and communities must be empowered to identify their own needs and priorities for action and must develop strategies and tactics to allow them to put such priorities into action. One way of doing this is through Rapid Participatory Appraisal (RPA) approaches. Within RPA multidisciplinary approaches and intersectoral working for health are of key importance. So too is the role of the user/client in evaluating and planning healthcare.

What is Rapid Participatory Appraisal (RPA)?

Rapid Participatory Appraisal (RPA) is a research approach that has been applied to a number of settings and covers a variety of methods and techniques (Scrimshaw and Hutardo, 1988; Thies and Grady, 1991; Ong *et al.*, 1991; Shamian and Kupe, 1993; Varkevissor, 1993). Used within the context of health it can provide an insight into a community's perspective of its priority needs which is a picture of the strength of feeling rather than a quantifiable measure of a particular problem. RPA also provides fast relevant information for decision-makers on priority issues they may face in service settings. It is very much a team exercise and one that is always carried out with the community in identifying needs and formulating action plans. It is primarily a tool for participatory diagnosis and planning, culminating in the formulation of action plans jointly with managers who have the resources to meet the community needs identified.

RPA can increase a community's access to health information, improve its access to health services, and empower it to influence and develop services to meet its health needs. It can estimate the strength of feeling of a community and offer an insight into what the problems are, as well as helping to define the health and social needs of deprived communities by:

- involving local people in identifying needs and service shortfalls and strengthening the principles of equity
- providing detailed knowledge of local areas and communities in the field with greater speed than conventional methods of analysis

- illustrating close working relationships with colleagues in other agencies operating in the same area, such as community and voluntary agencies and co-operating for a more accurate collection of information
- identifying of local health issues and better access for local people both to named professionals directly providing services and also to known managers and planners of services
- providing a focus for identifying health concerns linked to economic and social inequalities such as unemployment, poverty, social exclusion and poor housing
- creating a relevant, coordinated inter-agency response and multidisciplinary planning with room for flexibility and innovation
- demonstrating the significance of user involvement as a way of equalizing access to and experience of healthcare as a contribution to equalizing chances
- placing emphasis on producing timely insights (immediate and intermediate effects), hypotheses (theory generating), rather than final truths or fixed recommendations.

The key features are that a team is formed, involving people from various local organizations, to collect data from epidemiological information, local studies, existing written records, and more qualitatively and quantitatively from the communities themselves, and by using the opinions of a range of informants and their observations about the neighbourhood. The informants should be chosen for their knowledge of the local community and may include GPs, teachers, nurses, health visitors, midwives and social workers, police, voluntary and community leaders. Such information collection is based on the concept of 'triangulation', i.e. data from one source can be checked and validated by several other sources (see Figure 10.1). The approach does not lose

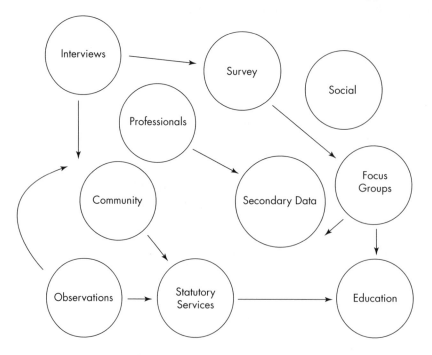

Figure 10.1 The concept of triangulation

concepts of validity and scientific rigour. Indeed, using data from a variety of sources and methods can strengthen needs assessment in that if all data point in the same direction it may be reasonably assumed that the insights gained are valid and valuable (see Chapter 5).

Once areas of concern have been identified, the information is fed back into the community in order for it to identify priorities for action. This technique strengthens the principles of equity, participation, ensures a concept of holistic health and attempts to investigate the totality of the core characteristics of success which may contribute to the individual's and/or the community's health (see Chapter 7, Stage 6). The information gathered can form a baseline for assessing the impact of interventions and services on the improvement of health and social need within the community. The process can also outline and identify available resources within the community that could address those needs. For community development, it is important to build upon a community's strengths rather than on its deficits.

Annett and Rifkin (1988) advocate the use of an information pyramid in collecting and analysing data in Rapid Participatory Appraisal exercises. As Figure 10.2 illustrates, the pyramid covers nine aspects used to assess community health needs.

- The base level contains information about community structures, interests and capacity to act – the main diagnosis and planning processes
- The second level has information about the environmental, socio-economic, disease and disability features – illustrating the potential but also any barriers which may exist for community improvements
- The third level covers the provision, accessibility and acceptability of health, environmental and social services. It forms the basis for the direct evaluation of effectiveness of present provision and provides indicators for change
- The final level concentrates on government policies – national, regional and local – about health improvements for deprived areas.

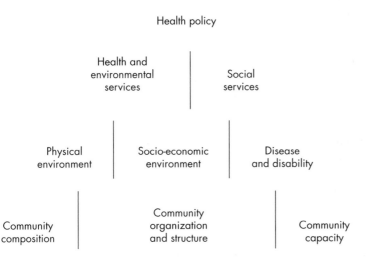

Figure 10.2 Information profile. Adapted from Annett and Rifkin (1988)

A community case study

Poverty and deprivation are determined by a number of complex and often inter-relating factors such as socio-economic status, lifestyle, geographical location, age, gender and community background, but primarily they are caused by high rates of unemployment and low incomes. The majority of people living on and below the poverty line are women (Oppenheim and Harker, 1996) (see Chapter 2).

The case study was carried out in an area with a population of around 7,000 that is recognized as being one of the most concentrated areas of deprivation in the UK (Lazenbatt *et al.*, 1999). Statistics paint a grim picture as the area scores poorly on all the census variables used to compile indices of deprivation, for example, the Townsend Index (Townsend *et al.*, 1988). Based on the 1991 Census statistics, it has a Townsend score of 9.84 ranking it the fifth most disadvantaged ward in the country. The association between poverty and ill health is well established, so it comes as no surprise that the health profile of the residents is poor. The standardized mortality ratio (SMR) for all causes of death under 65 is 164, where 100 is the average for the more affluent electoral wards in the wider area. There are particularly high rates of respiratory disease (SMR 156), heart disease (SMR 154), cancers (SMR 153) and injury (SMR 213).

The area has a younger population structure than other surrounding wards and has the highest proportion of births to teenage and single mothers, as well as one of the highest rates of infant mortality. It has some of the lowest rates of immunization and a high rate of community members suffering from long-term illness. Unemployment is one of the most serious problems facing the area today (INCORE, 1997). The result of this serious unemployment problem for both male and female residents is a situation of high dependency and low-average household income levels. Non-ownership of a car limits access to healthcare, especially primary care. Better access could reduce the number of avoidable hospitalizations and the number of community members using casualty departments as local health centres. The picture is predictable and fits well into a stereotype of disadvantaged inner-city neighbourhoods. Statistics such as these are a starting point for health promotion work, but it can be difficult to develop a comprehensive assessment of needs on this basis.

Aims and objectives

The aims of this case study are to demonstrate the use of Rapid Participatory Appraisal in:

- gaining insights into women's health and social needs which are based on their own and other agencies' perspectives over a short period of time
- assessing whether there are sufficient and correctly designed services to address health and social problems within the community
- assessing whether there are barriers that prevent certain groups from accessing services
- translating these findings into action; and
- establishing an on-going relationship between service providers, voluntary organizations and local communities.

The objectives are to:

- raise awareness of women's health needs in the community
- develop collaborative working on a partnership basis with statutory and voluntary agencies and also community groups with an interest in tackling health inequalities
- train and resource a network of lay people interested in health issues
- ensure the provision of services and support specifically for women
- disseminate health information in an acceptable form.

Method

There are seven stages in Rapid Participatory Appraisal:

1   Define Rapid Participatory Appraisal – selecting the RPA team
2   Define what information is needed
3   Decide how to obtain information
        involve the community in RPA
        key informant interviews
        observation
        secondary documents
4   Collect information
5   Analyse information
6   Prioritization of needs
7   Feedback
8   Conclusions
9   Programme of change

Stage 1: Define Rapid Participatory Appraisal (RPA): Selecting the RPA team

Remember that RPA attempts to investigate elements which contribute to an individual's and a community's health. From the list of features already identified under the heading of What is Rapid Participatory Appraisal (RPA)?, we can now select those which have the most useful bearing on the local community. For the community, RPA needs assessment has a number of key advantages in that it can:

- provide a detailed knowledge of the local area and community
- illustrate close working relationships with colleagues in other agencies, operating in the same area, such as local authorities and voluntary agencies co-operating for more accurate collection of information
- lead to the identification of local health issues and better access for local women both to named professionals directly providing services and also to known managers and planners of services
- provide a focus for identifying women's health concerns linked to economic and social inequalities such as low income, unemployment, poverty and poor housing
- involve local women in identifying needs and service shortfalls

- create a relevant, coordinated inter-agency response
- demonstrate the significance of user involvement as a way of equalizing access to and experience of healthcare as a contribution to equalizing chances.

It is essential to define the parameters of the needs assessment and to take a positive RPA approach by collecting baseline data about the problems or needs, rather than about the solution. The optimal solution may vary in nature, depending on the information yielded by baseline data. It may not always be a service, but may be some form of community action to remove or change the root cause of the problem.

Using a workshop format, a team was brought together who were capable of looking at the different aspects of holistic health. The RPA team represented members of different organizations and disciplinary backgrounds as well as resource holders. This was somewhat larger than the typical RPA team, which usually consists of 10–12 people. Nevertheless, it was thought essential that the various team members were assembled to agree the main objectives of the RPA exercise. During this initial workshop the team set the direction for the project and a decision was made to assess women's health needs within the community.

Team membership

Board Secretary and Acting Head of
   Education for the Royal College of
   Nursing (RCN)
Director of Nursing – Community Trust
Voluntary organization – Lifestart
Health centre manager
GP from Health Centre
Coordinator from Health Centre
District nurse
Health visitor
Nurse practitioner

Chairman, British Medical Association
Community assistant in Health Centre
Community worker
Community housing facilitator
Community Women's Forum
Community Women's Group members
Carer and Women's Forum member
University lecturer and researcher
Nurse lecturer from Royal College of Nursing
   (RCN)
Professor of Mental Health

It was at times difficult to organize meetings with the larger group of team members as they were often senior managers and professionals who were extremely busy. However, they were convinced of the appropriateness and usefulness of the RPA in terms of delivering short-term goals. A sub-team was therefore created and it contained members from the universities, the RCN, the community and nursing professionals. As the sub-team could not work full-time, the Rapid Participatory Appraisal was undertaken over a four-month period with each team member contributing four hours per week.

Stage 2: Decide what information is needed

In a one-day workshop the team made decisions about what sort of information needed to be obtained, how it would best be collected and what information could be extracted from written and observational records. Information is usually collected on all nine aspects of the pyramid (Figure 10.2) and data is collected from three main sources: existing written records, interviews with a range of key informants and interviews and surveys with the community.

The objectives of the workshop were to:

- Define the area of focus – women's health needs in the community
- Define work programme and timetable
- Agree an understanding of the main context and limitations of RPA
- Set up focus groups to generate questions
- Conduct a survey with and by the community
- Analyse existing data
- Set priorities.

Stage 3: Decide how to obtain information

During the initial workshop existing documentation was analysed and gaps in information identified. A protocol was designed to set out the specific purpose of the needs assessment and to identify key informants as listed below. From this extended list of potential informants, the RPA team interviewed local health service professionals, health visitors, midwives, teachers, social workers, voluntary organizations and community representatives. Although this data source can enhance understanding of an issue or problem, it is important to bear in mind that key informants may have their own biases and prejudices that might emerge during the interview.

Key informants

Government officials	Social workers
Social and health service personnel	Legal profession
Health visitors	Media networks
Midwives	Community leaders: women's groups,
Patients	support groups, community
GPs	organizations
Teachers	Voluntary agencies
Pharmacists	

Within the workshop setting the team decided that information from the community should be elicited by using a focus group and a community health survey which was to be conducted by community members (see Appendix 1 for the Questionnaire). The community survey covered aspects of women's health and included areas such as:

Demographic details   marital status, family composition, age, employment, social class, education, transport, housing, benefits etc.

Lifestyle   smoking, smoking and pregnancy, alcohol, alcohol and pregnancy, drugs – prescription and recreational etc.

Mental health   anxiety, depression and stress, coping mechanisms, psychiatric treatment, support mechanisms etc.

Nutrition and leisure   eating habits, weight, leisure time, physical activities, exercise, etc.

Sexual health   sex education, family planning, sexually transmitted disease etc.

Reproductive health   pregnancy, antenatal and postnatal care, breastfeeding, social support, parenting skills, gynaecological history, screening – smears, mammograms, menopause, HRT etc.

Women and disability   physical, psychological or leaning disability

Women and caring   relationship, employment, support, financial difficulties, health effects

Women and violence   abuse, rape, health problems, support etc.

Women and children   children's disability, behavioural problems, physical illness, accidents, schooling, development, adoption etc.

Education and communication   media, newspapers, social cohesion in community, educational facilities etc.

Access to services   primary care team, clinics, services, barriers, needs etc.

Self assessment of health   ill health, consulting GP, prescriptions, etc.

Available secondary data and sources of written information (detailed below) from the area were also scrutinized and plans were drawn up for the fieldwork, which took the form of supplementary interviews with key informants and the community survey.

Sources of written information

Census statistics

Planning records

Surveys already undertaken in the area

Government agencies

Professional organizations

University publications

Health providers' reports

Reports of studies undertaken within universities

Historical records

Regional health statistics

Internet search

Hospital records

Studies and surveys by other agencies

Records relating to housing, environment, social services etc.

Table 10.1 Indicators of deprivation in the community

Robson Index	Urban Institute Index
Pensioners lacking central heating	Unemployment
Overcrowding	Women economically inactive
Children in low-earner households	Dependent population (<16 and >65)
17/18-year-olds without qualifications	Share of population in
Unemployment	socio-economic classes 4 and 5

In most cases data already existed which were relevant to the community such as census materials, reports from both statutory and voluntary agencies, as well as projects carried out by professionals. Without information on local deprivation levels and the health and social costs of poverty for women and families, the RPA team were unlikely to be able to evaluate effectiveness of current strategies or make judgments about how they should be responding to poverty and health issues. To obtain some understanding of the patterns of deprivation, it was possible to look at the distribution of particular social problems using scores on the Robson Index and the Urban Institute Index (Table 10.1).

Stage 4: Collect information

The sub-team undertook the focus groups and training sessions with ten community representatives who had agreed to undertake the community survey. These community representatives were paid for their work from funding obtained through Glaxo Wellcome. It was decided that 20 members of the community would be interviewed in a focus group setting. This was led by a person skilled in facilitating focus group discussion. A semi-structured interview schedule was prepared, which took the form of a broad framework of issues adapted from the pyramid in Figure 10.2 (see Appendix 2). The topics covered community composition, socio-economic and housing issues, access to services, etc. The goal was to elicit the community views through a guided questioning route and for the sub-team to emerge from the focus group with a deeper understanding of the 'community's' priority health and social need issues. The team made an inventory of all the different sources of information and defined a framework for analysis, based on the approach of 'triangulation', which allows the researcher to look at one issue from various perspectives (see Chapter 5).

For the survey, a target group of 100 households was defined as a sub-group of the community. The ten community representatives undertaking the survey selected a number of households and carried out the interviews. Consent was obtained from the respondents and they were given written material outlining the purpose of the survey. The interviews were carried out in a relaxed, informal manner, and members of the family were often drawn into the discussion and questioning. The community approach allowed discussion of the same question from several angles.

Stage 5: Analyse information

Most of the data collected from the key informants, through the focus groups, and from the secondary documents was not readily quantifiable and therefore analysis required a systematic approach using content analysis. It was important to assess the data by identifying categories, sorting answers and interpreting the findings. However, the data collected through the community survey was much more quantifiable and allowed for statistical analysis. All the data were reduced to categories within which specific priorities were established. Each category was placed on an index card along with the appropriate priorities listed. The main categories were:

- Physical environment
- Disease
- Mental health issues
- Lifestyle
- Access to health services
- Socio-economic issues

Before assessing the community's view about priorities the team first ranked the items themselves to provide a comparison of their opinions with those of the community. Moreover, the team tried to rank order on the basis of observation and what they understood the community view to be. Following this and during a feedback meeting with the community the RPA team asked them to place these priority lists in rank order. This started a two-way discussion about the opportunities for change during which the RPA team learned more about the main concerns of the community, the limitations of statutory services and the need to prioritize problems. Following this all the data on each category was reduced to a number of statements describing key needs for the community. A group of local GPs was also asked to rank-order the priority list. This priority setting exercise with the three groups allowed a comparison to be made between them. In other words, it was ascertained whether the priorities chosen by the community members were of equal value to those chosen by the GPs and the RPA team. The comparisons could then be drawn using a statistical comparison or weighted approach.

A nonparametric statistical method used in RPA is Kendall's coefficient of concordance. This is a statistical technique used to examine the level of agreement between each of a set of 'judges' (i.e. any individual who is invited to participate in the community priority setting). These individuals have to rank-order their priorities in each of the selected categories. Their scores are compared with each other within a category, and the lowest score denotes the highest priority.

The three sets of rankings were analysed separately to assess the extent of agreements amongst the 'judges' by utilizing Kendall's coefficient of concordance. The analysis of the rank order data employing non-parametric statistical techniques was conducted through the university. The mean rankings are presented in Table 10.2.

With respect to environmental issues, the GPs, the RPA team and the community all had political boundaries and problems with access to services because of this at the top of the list. The highest priority for the community was the problem of transport due in many cases to poor car availability. With respect to disease the community considered breast cancer the main issue and they were very close in their judgment to the GPs who

Table 10.2 Categories of women's health needs and priority issues (mean ranks)

	Team GP view (n=6)	Team view of community (n=6)	Community view (n=25)
Physical environment			
Political boundaries	1.9	1.5	1.8
Transport	2.0	1.8	1.6
Lack of facilities	3.0	2.9	2.2
Disease			
Breast cancer	2.1	2.0	1.7
Cervical cancer	2.4	2.9	2.4
Heart disease	1.5	2.1	2.3
Mental health issues			
Depression	2.1	3.1	3.2
Stress	2.7	2.9	2.9
Anxiety and fear	3.1	2.8	2.7
Lifestyle			
Smoking	2.1	3.1	3.2
Alcohol problems	3.0	3.1	4.4
Access to services			
Baby clinic	3.4	2.7	2.4
Well woman clinic	2.8	3.2	2.3
Asthma clinic	1.9	1.9	3.2
Socio-economic			
Poverty	2.4	1.9	1.6
Unemployment	2.2	1.8	1.6
Low pay	3.0	2.8	2.7

saw also breast cancer and cervical cancer as priorities, although their highest priority was heart disease. While poverty itself was difficult to address directly, as it was closely associated with high regional levels of unemployment and a dearth of job opportunities, the community felt that alleviating poverty remained high on their agenda as well as a focus on unemployment. The RPA team and the GP group also registered unemployment their highest priority. With respect to access to services, the GP group and the RPA team felt that an asthma clinic was necessary for the area while the community felt a well woman clinic was highest on their priority list. The highest priority of the GP group with respect to mental health issues was the level of depression, while anxiety and fear were placed highest for community and the RPA team. Smoking was the highest priority within lifestyle issues for all the groups.

Stage 6: Prioritization of needs

Survey results

The community survey results were analysed using the Statistical Package for the Social Sciences (SPSSPC). This is a comprehensive, integrated computer programme for managing, analysing and displaying data (see *SPSS – PC User's Guide*). Eighty-five women in the community answered the survey and this was a response rate of 85%. The mean age was 33 years and ages ranged from 22 to 54 years. Almost a quarter of the women were employed (22%), but many were in part-time work with low incomes. The results of the survey are discussed in line with the categories of health needs and priorities already established.

Physical environment

The survey illustrated that there is limited access to efficient and cheap transport (75%), there are problems with political boundaries (86%), and lack of leisure facilities in the area (45%). Women were concerned about the lack of crèche and pre-school facilities and also the safety of their children in the streets due to lack of play areas for toddlers and young children. Women in the community suffer from considerable isolation which in many cases is exacerbated by relatively poor car availability especially for elderly women and women with young children. The 'troubles' still have an effect on the community as there are political boundaries within the area, which means that access to some services is difficult for the women as they have to cross these boundaries to attend baby and well women clinics.

Disease

The results show that a strikingly high percentage of women (31%) suffer from breast and cervical cancer (age range 31–53 years). However, it is interesting to note that 70% of the women had been screened for cancer with both mammograms and smears thanks to the Action Cancer mobile screening unit which came to the health centre the previous year. Diabetes, raised blood pressure, respiratory disease, and arthritis were also identified as health problems.

Mental health issues

The survey shows that a significant number of women in the area suffer serious problems with stress (62%), depression (53%), anxiety/worry (24%). Depression was highest among those women who were looking after a family and were living in an unemployed household. Primary healthcare teams showed considerable awareness of the 'fragile' mental state of many of these women and how this was related to high rates of repeat prescriptions for sleeping tablets (21%), valium (25%), anti-depressants (42%) and recreational drugs such as cannabis (12%).

Almost three-quarters (73%) of the women felt stressed. The reasons for stress for women within this specific community were the political situation (87%), fear of crime (52%), financial worries (45%) and long-term and generational unemployment (41%). There was a perception among residents that certain streets had paedophiles who were regularly taunting young girls and boys and trying to buy their favours. This was extremely distressing for mothers and they were anxious about the effect of this on their younger children. They were also concerned for teenagers, as recreational drugs were freely available in the community. Time and again they voiced a sense of outrage that so little was being done about both of these issues.

The stress of these situations for the people living in the area cannot be under-estimated. Health visitors and social workers in the community are only too aware of these problems. Most women sought support from their GPs for stress and this was evidenced by the high number of repeat prescriptions for tranquillizers and anti-depressants (67%). This associated stress and anxiety made the women want to move out of the troubled neighbourhood as soon as they could to the further detriment of social cohesion and stability in the area.

Lifestyle

The survey showed that almost three-quarters of the women (72%) were smokers and considered it to be a serious problem for themselves and their families, and 58% of these smokers rated it as a serious health problem for the community as a whole. Their smoking habits were sustained despite knowledge of the health risks of smoking. Women in the community were aware that they faced extra health problems such as increases in the risk of stroke and heart disease as well as cervical cancer. However, they were unaware that in pregnancy it can adversely affect the development of the foetus and that the menopause can occur earlier in women who smoke and may result in the onset of osteoporosis. Smoking was seen as a stress reduction strategy for many women who smoked (58%).

In contrast to their smoking behaviour, drinking habits were well within safe limits. While smoking formed an integral part of their daily routine, drinking alcohol was an activity for one or two evenings a week. Even under stress most women claimed that they would not turn to drink as a coping strategy. However, a small number (8%) stated that they would be more likely to drink heavily if under stress and they needed to calm their nerves.

Access to services

Most of the comments about primary care services were favourable. However, two-thirds (65%) of the women felt that there were particular problems of access, and barriers to services and facilities particularly for women and their children. In many cases access to their health centre was difficult for those with no car. A number of women mentioned the shortage of childcare facilities. The survey showed that 24% of the women had attended casualty during the last twelve months and 80% had seen a GP. The main suggestions for improvements of services were a well woman clinic, baby clinic, stress management and more health promoting classes to cover smoking cessation and healthy eating.

Socio-economic issues

Eighty per cent of the women had fears and insecurity with regard to work and money. The women with children spoke of the difficulties involved in getting jobs that fitted with school hours and of finding appropriate and affordable childcare. Many were struggling to make ends meet. Women were also concerned with providing for their children, both in terms of necessities such as good food, clothes and shoes but also in terms of 'treats' like days out and holidays. Another source of stress was financial insecurity. The financially insecure reported serious problems with buying food and paying household bills. More elderly women expressed most concern about heating bills, incurred by the need to maintain a high level of heating because of a sick or disabled person in the household. They felt that they were in a cycle of fuel poverty. The combination of low income, debts and the inability to afford certain major items was clearly having a negative effect on the women's quality of life.

Summary

It is clear from the survey that problems with physical health are connected with a wide range of factors relating to stress, environmental conditions, political boundaries, financial circumstances, dietary and smoking habits and lack of health promotion in the area. Concern among GPs in the area is about coronary heart disease and other smoking-related health problems such as cancer, respiratory and circulatory diseases and is consistent with the available statistics. However, for the women in the community there is perhaps a rather different perception of the relative importance of heart disease as opposed to respiratory disease and breast and cervical cancer. Particular complex problems were highlighted by the younger woman with children such as financial difficulties, problems of access to work (due to lack of affordable childcare facilities), children with asthma, poor diet and smoking, isolation and lack of parenting skills leading to worry and depression. In several cases this was exacerbated by several young women having serious health problems such as breast and cervical cancer. One woman stated that: 'Cancer is like the common cold in the community'.

Stage 7: Feedback

To make RPA transparent and accountable, feedback had to be given to the community, both about the process and the outcome (see Chapter 9, Stages 8 and 9). A written report about the process and the priority listings was distributed to the community. Public meetings or smaller gatherings were arranged to discuss the findings of this rapid participatory appraisal exercise. It was important at this stage to build up the community's capacity by:

- providing mechanisms to increase their ability to cope with stress
- creating strong social support systems and networks
- providing a sense of wellbeing.

This case study illustrates the dual approach to problem solving as the team tried to define the action that could be taken by the community and action that statutory services could undertake to support the community. Rather than determining priorities and strategies, the role of professionals is one of empowering the community to help itself.

Stage 8: Conclusions

The results show that, despite intensive dialogue between community and professionals, the understanding that professionals have regarding the community's problems are mediated by their resource restrictions. This is not to dismiss professional judgment but rather to illustrate the complexities involved in sharing information and understanding needs. The Rapid Participatory Appraisal team did not feel that they could accept the community's word totally, since there are issues that need further debate and their priorities cannot always be taken at face value. To illustrate this more fully, the community did not mention smoking cessation as an important issue for women's health, although evidence-based healthcare suggests that stopping smoking has important benefits for women in particular. It would therefore be impossible both from a professional and government point of view to drop this as a key priority, so on-going debate with the community is vitally important.

The case study emphasizes the problems of urban deprivation, placing the problems of political boundaries and unemployment as high priorities. The RPA team feel, that as well as exposing the level and extent of poverty in the area, RPA has given them a greater insight into unmet health and social needs, such as:

- poor nursery provision for the under-fives
- lack of safe play areas
- fuel poverty for the elderly person
- women's high dependence on prescription drugs such as valium and anti-depressants
- lack of access to specific services due to political boundaries.

For many low-income families there is little hope that their circumstances will change for the better in the near future. However, the provision of services such as well women and baby clinics and stress management classes that can assist families to cope with the material and health effects of breadline living seems to offer an important improvement.

Smoking for women in this area is a serious problem not only to them but also to their children and families. Evidence from Graham's (1988) research into women and smoking indicates that the capacity for people living on low income to respond to health education and to change their behaviour is often limited. Graham's research is important as it leads us to make the link between stress and smoking. Wilkinson argues that higher levels of behavioural risk-taking among poorer people reflect high levels of chronic stress rather than ignorance of the health risks associated with smoking (Wilkinson 1996, p. 188). He suggests that studies which focus on the links between material disadvantage and poor health, among those living on low incomes are missing the point:

> To feel depressed, cheated, bitter, desperate, vulnerable, frightened, angry, worried about debt, to feel devalued, useless, helpless, hopeless, anxious, isolated: these feelings can dominate people's whole experience of life, colouring their experience of everything else. It is the chronic stress arising from these feelings which does the damage. It is the social feelings which matter, not exposure to a supposedly toxic material environment.
>
> (Wilkinson, 1996, p. 215)

Stage 9: Programme of change

It is a very daunting task to create a coherent needs assessment methodology built on both objective and subjective definitions of need which will take into account community diversity as well as the central issue of inequality. This case study shows that RPA which can bring together the professional view and the users' view (which focuses on the consequences of disease and social need in everyday life) is an appropriate method to use. However, needs assessment cannot be divorced from issues of effectiveness and cost-effectiveness, priority setting and the uneasy balance between individual or population health gain.

The attraction of the method is its flexibility. The case study was undertaken in four months which is rapid in comparison with other research and community needs projects. The intersectoral multi-professional and multi-agency public health approach to health was essential in the dialogue with the community, as it was obvious that they defined health in a very holistic way to include environmental, political and socio-economic issues. It showed that access to data sources such as census and epidemiological information requires the addition of more qualitative and quantitative data concerned with the communities' views of their health needs. Together these formed a powerful baseline for assessing the impact of services on the improvement of the life and health of populations and communities. In the community, where health and social services management is largely localized, the input from the community in planning and evaluating services can be even more focused through using RPA techniques alongside more conventional quantitative methods.

In RPA a small number of actions which involve the community and one or two agencies can be agreed within a short time (usually six months), although, some key priorities cannot be addressed because they are too large scale and are beyond the scope of the organizations involved. However, even on a more modest scale regular evaluation of progress is necessary and a mechanism has to be found or devised to carry out these evaluations, which can be established through the community. Agreement has to be reached about the criteria for success and the way in which certain actions are brought to a close. RPA has a limited life and after a certain period of time the community is likely to have evolved as a result of wider social and economic changes.

As expected, there was considerable difference between the individual professional and voluntary groups and the community. Although the RPA team found variations between the priorities of local people, on the one hand, and professionals and GPs, on the other, differences between professional groups appeared to be more significant. Such differences emphasize the importance of inter-agency and multidisciplinary responses to health and social problems and the need to encourage participation by local communities in order to maximize the agreement between the priorities of professionals and those of local people. The findings suggest that many single agency or single professional responses are likely to result in measures that are out of tune with residents' own perceptions of needs and priorities.

The results show that, despite intensive dialogue between community and professionals, the proactive measures of professionals are mediated by their inability to alleviate poverty and unemployment. The primary healthcare professionals did explain the limitations of their influence on inequalities in health and the budgetary constraints placed upon them to extend their services.

Immediate outcomes

- The needs assessment was generated and conducted within the community and allowed local people to work in partnership with professionals in the statutory services and voluntary organizations, thus creating a 'culture of participation' in relation to the planning and delivery of services.
- Within primary healthcare, lack of planning time and the pressure to respond to the immediate needs of patients mean that local needs assessments are given low priority. This case study shows that RPA provides a structure to elicit and learn from local opinions. Using local women to do the research has many advantages.
- A health forum is being established following this RPA to include members of statutory groups, voluntary and community groups etc. It is hoped that this will allow permanent dialogue between the community and professionals in which action plans might be instigated and evaluated, as many of the important health and social needs could not be met by health services alone.
- The RPA team have been able to transfer skills and information to local women so that they can work to secure resources for their community. Outside funding is now being sought from the National Lottery Poverty and Community Programmes for the creation of a Lay Health Worker Project in the area. It is hoped that local people will be recruited to establish support groups for frail elderly people, those who suffer from depression, for young inexperienced postnatal mothers and for unemployed individuals. Local workers could also work in health promotion activities such as smoking cessation and better eating campaigns. The community has been centrally involved in writing bids, thus building up their knowledge of project proposals and negotiation with funding bodies.

Intermediate outcomes

- The role of the health centre manager is seen as central in harnessing local efforts as she is most accessible and in touch with the community. She has arranged to meet several people including GPs to formulate intermediate steps, to support new ideas, and to act as a link with statutory and voluntary services. As a result of the RPA exercise, liaison between health, social services and voluntary organizations was strengthened both at community and managerial level.
- One GP has responded to feedback from the community and has identified a need for a nurse practitioner in the health centre. The post is now being advertised and the role of the nurse practitioner will be to help the women in the community by providing a well woman clinic, stress management classes, smoking cessation groups, alternative therapies and improving the running of the local practice. The community Trust is also introducing a baby clinic and asthma clinic into the health centre.

Longer-term outcomes

- Baseline measures have been collected that are linked to longer-term outcomes such as rates of smoking cessation, improvements in housing conditions, increased child immunization, increased screening rates for women, increased access to health services etc. Such information will allow a comparison of these issues at a later time.

Success Indicators	Needs Assessment

1 APPROACHES/PARTNERSHIPS

Health alliances
The challenge for improving public health goes far beyond imparting information about healthy lifestyles, preventative care, or even quality of care. At its roots, the challenge for public health calls for consumers to participate as full partners in the healthcare system, actively responsible for their own health maintenance and vigilant in demanding quality and cost-effectiveness. The principles of a community approach to a problem involve the participation in and ownership of agendas by all involved. Traditional methods of health assessment use a more directive, top-down approach: experts define the problem, and then suggest solutions.

Inter-agency
Rapid Participatory Appraisal can create a relevant, coordinated inter-agency response and multidisciplinary planning with room for flexibility and innovation when defining health and social needs of deprived communities.

Multidisciplinary
Multidisciplinary approaches and intersectoral working for health are of key importance within Rapid Participatory Appraisal as is the role of the user in evaluating and planning healthcare.

2 TOOLS (METHODS)

Evaluation
All evaluations require some form of baseline information or needs assessment measures to allow achievement to be measured against a yardstick or to act as a benchmark. One of the key questions within an evaluation process is how resources should be distributed, reflecting local needs. Traditionally, health services plan distribution on the basis of service use, but if needs are considered to incorporate felt, but not unmet needs, then this approach falls short.

Research
Rapid Participatory Appraisal is a research approach that has been applied to a number of settings and covers a variety of methods and techniques (both qualitative and

quantitative). It is a tool for participatory diagnosis and planning, culminating in the formulation of action plans jointly with managers who have the resources to meet the needs identified. This analysis of the area, together with evidence drawn from the experience of the front-line staff and others about health prevention and promotion, provides valuable additional information in their assessment of health and social need.

Needs assessment

The equitable provision of healthcare must begin with a systematic assessment of needs of target groups and the need to set priorities in order to provide resources in the most efficient way to meet the needs of populations and different social groups. A key feature of RPA is that it can provide the structure to develop an in-depth profile of the designated area. It can identify factors influencing the health of the population, and highlight smaller areas and target groups facing particular obstacles to securing good health and social wellbeing and access to adequate services.

3 RESOURCES

Setting

The case study was carried out in a community, with a population of around 7,000, and recognized as being one of the most concentrated areas of deprivation in the UK. Levels of deprivation have been compounded by the heavy burden suffered by the area from the Northern Ireland troubles. According to *The Costs of the Troubles Survey* (INCORE, 1997) the area has experienced some of the highest number of deaths in the UK. This combination of violence and deprivation has had a crucial impact on health and the quality of life in the area, particularly for women.

Delivery agent

Using a workshop format a small team was brought together capable of looking at the different aspects of holistic health and representing resource holders from various organizations. A typical RPA team consists of 10–12 people from different organizations and disciplinary backgrounds. It is essential that the various team members are brought together to agree the main objectives of the RPA exercise. Profiling and monitoring the impact of poverty and deprivation were seen as essential to any evaluation. Without such information on local deprivation levels and the health and social costs of poverty for women and families, evaluators are unlikely to be able to evaluate effectiveness of current strategies or make judgements about how they should be responding to poverty and health issues.

Training delivery agent

The team divided into a smaller sub-team with members from the community, the university and nursing. The sub-team undertook a training session with ten community representatives who had agreed to undertake the community survey. For the survey, a target group of 100 households was defined as a sub-group of the community. The ten community representatives undertaking the survey selected a number of households and carried out the interviews. Consent was obtained from the respondents and they were given written material outlining purpose of the survey. The interviews were carried out in a relaxed, informal manner, and members of the family were often drawn into the discussion and questioning. The community approach allowed discussion of the same question from several angles.

4 INDIVIDUAL/COMMUNITY

Holistic health
Health within the boundaries of inequalities is based on a total holistic concept including understanding the person's physical, mental, social, and environmental wellbeing, thus moving outside the narrow medical definition. Rapid Participatory Appraisal strengthens the principles of equity, participation and ensures a total concept of health.

Culture
Poverty, deprivation and social exclusion are determined by a number of complex and often inter-relating factors such as socio-economic status, lifestyle, geographical location, age, gender and community background, but primarily they are caused by high rates of unemployment, and low incomes. The majority of people living on and below the poverty line are women.

Community development
Once areas of concern have been identified, the information is fed back into the community in order for them to identify priorities for action. This approach strengthens the principles of equity, participation, ensures a concept of holistic health and attempts to investigate the totality of the core characteristics of success which may contribute to the individual's and/or the community's health. The information gathered can form a baseline for assessing the impact of interventions and services on the improvement of health and social need within the community. The process should also outline and identify available resources within the community that could address those needs. For community development to occur, it is important to build upon a community's strengths rather than on its deficits.

Empowerment
Tackling inequalities by empowering individuals and communities requires communities to identify their own needs and priorities for action by developing strategies and tactics to meet them. Rapid Participatory Appraisal can increase access to health information, improve access to health services, and empower service users to influence and develop services to meet their health needs. It can tell the strength of feeling of a community and offer an insight into what the problems are as well as help define the health and social needs in deprived communities.

APPENDIX 1

A questionnaire from the Women's Community Health Survey

Demographic details

Age   ☐ 1

1.   Marital status of the respondent
         Married   ☐ 1
         Divorced/legally separated   ☐ 2
         Separated   ☐ 3
         Single (alone)   ☐ 4
         Widowed   ☐ 5
         Single (steady relationship)   ☐ 6
         Single (living partner)   ☐ 7
         Married (living apart)   ☐ 8
         Exclusion Order   ☐ 9

2.   Family composition (people living in the house)
         Partner/husband   ☐ 1
         Son(s)   ☐ 2
         Daughter(s)   ☐ 3
         Living alone   ☐ 4
         Mother   ☐ 5
         Father   ☐ 6
         Relative   ☐ 7
         Other   ☐ 8
     Please specify the number of people living in the house   ☐ 9

3.   Age groups
         No of children aged 0–5 years   ☐ 1
         No of children aged 6–17 years   ☐ 2
         No of adults aged 18–45 years   ☐ 3
         No of adults aged 45–60 years   ☐ 4
         No of adults aged over 60 years   ☐ 5

4.   Employment status
         Full-time   ☐ 1
         Part-time   ☐ 2
         Unemployed   ☐ 3
         Engaged in home duties   ☐ 4
         Student   ☐ 5
         Retired   ☐ 6
         Ill/disabled   ☐ 7
         Have you ever been employed?   ☐ 8
         Generations unemployed   ☐ 9

Other   ☐ 10
(Specify: _____)

6.   Employment status of partner/husband
      Full-time   ☐ 1
      Part-time   ☐ 2
      Unemployed   ☐ 3
      Engaged in home duties   ☐ 4
      Student   ☐ 5
      Retired   ☐ 6
      Ill/disabled   ☐ 7
      Has he ever been employed?   ☐ 8
      Generations unemployed   ☐ 9
      Other   ☐ 10
      (Specify: _____)

7.   Social class
      Professional   ☐ 1
      Managerial/technical   ☐ 2
      Skilled – non-manual   ☐ 3
      Skilled – manual   ☐ 4
      Partly skilled   ☐ 5
      Unskilled   ☐ 6

8.   What level of education have you attained?
      Primary school 11+   ☐ 1
      Secondary school   ☐ 2
      GCSE/'O' Levels   ☐ 3
      GCSE/'A' Levels   ☐ 4
      Technical   ☐ 5
      BTEC   ☐ 6
      HND   ☐ 7
      Degree/university   ☐ 8
      None   ☐ 9
      Other   ☐ 10
      (Specify: _____)

9.   Car ownership   YES   NO
      Do you own a car   ☐ 1   ☐ 2
      Do you have access to a car   ☐ 1   ☐ 2
      Car provided by DHSS   ☐ 1   ☐ 2

10. What form of transport do you use most?
      Taxi   ☐ 1
      Bus   ☐ 2

Car   ☐ 3
Other   ☐ 4
(Specify: _____)

11. Type of housing
     Housing executive   ☐ 1
     Own your own house   ☐ 2
     Rented accommodation   ☐ 3
     Homeless   ☐ 4
     Sheltered accommodation   ☐ 5
     Residential accommodation   ☐ 6
     Other   ☐ 7
     (Specify: _____)

12. Thinking of your housing is it:
     Damp   ☐ 1
     Draughty   ☐ 2
     Centrally heated   ☐ 3
     Got a garden   ☐ 4
     Overcrowded   ☐ 5
     Safe place to live   ☐ 6

13. Are you receiving any benefits?
     Yes   ☐ 1
     No   ☐ 2

14. If yes, are they:
     Housing benefit   ☐ 1
     Sickness benefit   ☐ 2
     Attendance allowance   ☐ 3
     Disability allowance   ☐ 4
     Family income supplement   ☐ 5
     Others   ☐ 6
     (Specify: _____)

15. Are you exempt from prescription charges?
     Yes   ☐ 1
     No   ☐ 2
     Don't know   ☐ 3

16. Are you a member of an ethnic minority?
     Yes   ☐ 1
     No   ☐ 2

Lifestyle

1.   Which of the following statements is true for you?

I smoke cigarettes regularly   □ 1
(at least 1 per day every day)
I smoke cigarettes occasionally   □ 2
I am an ex-smoker   □ 3
I have never smoked   □ 4

                                                    Go to 6.

2.   How many cigarettes do you smoke?

1–5   □ 1
6–10   □ 2
11–19   □ 3
20 or more   □ 4

3.   Why do you usually smoke?

To be sociable   □ 1
To enjoy a cigarette   □ 2
To relax   □ 3
To cope with depression   □ 4
To cope with family stress   □ 5
To cope with work stress   □ 6
Feel addicted   □ 7
Other   □ 8
(Specify: _____)
Don't know   □ 8

4.   Would you like to give up smoking?

Yes   □ 1
No   □ 2
Don't know   □ 3

5.   If yes, have you contacted someone to help you to stop?

GP   □ 1
Nurse   □ 2
Chemist   □ 1
Hospital   □ 2
Self-help/support group   □ 1
Community group   □ 2
Voluntary group   □ 1
(Specify: _____)

6.   If you have ever been pregnant, did you smoke during any of the
pregnancies?

Yes   □ 1

No ☐ 2
Can't remember ☐ 3
Never been pregnant ☐ 4

7.   During any of these pregnancies did anyone advise you to stop?
       GP ☐ 1
       Nurse ☐ 2
       Midwife ☐ 3
       Pharmacist ☐ 4
       Physiotherapist ☐ 5
       Friends/family ☐ 6
       Self-help/support group ☐ 7
       Community group ☐ 8
       Voluntary group ☐ 9
       (Specify: _____)

8.   If you were to become pregnant in the future, would you smoke during the pregnancy?
       Yes ☐ 1
       No ☐ 2
       Don't know ☐ 3

9.   Could you tell me if you agree or disagree with the following statements?

	Agree	Disagree	Don't know
Smoking increases the risk of lung cancer	☐ 1	☐ 2	☐ 3
Smoking increases the risk of heart disease	☐ 1	☐ 2	☐ 3
Smoking increases the risk of bronchitis	☐ 1	☐ 2	☐ 3
If a pregnant woman smokes her unborn baby smokes	☐ 1	☐ 2	☐ 3
Passive smoking is dangerous to others in the family	☐ 1	☐ 2	☐ 3
Smoking increases the risk of childhood asthma	☐ 1	☐ 2	☐ 3
Smoking increases the risk of childhood infections	☐ 1	☐ 2	☐ 3
Smoking increases the risk of miscarriage	☐ 1	☐ 2	☐ 3

10.   Can you tell me which of the following describes you?
       A person who takes a drink ☐ 1
       An ex drinker ☐ 2
       A person who has never taken alcohol ☐ 3
       Go to 16

11.   How may times in the last 12 months have you been drunk?
       Never in the 12 months ☐ 1

Once or twice   ☐ 2
3–5 times in 12 months   ☐ 3
Once a month   ☐ 4
1–2 times a week   ☐ 5
2–4 times a week   ☐ 6
Every day   ☐ 7
Other times   ☐ 8
(Specify: _____)

12. Why do you usually drink?
     To be sociable   ☐ 1
     To enjoy a drink   ☐ 2
     To relax   ☐ 3
     To cope with depression   ☐ 4
     To cope with family stress   ☐ 5
     To cope with work stress   ☐ 6
     Other   ☐ 7
     (Specify: _____)
     Don't know   ☐ 8

13. If you were ever pregnant, did you drink alcohol during the pregnancy?
     Yes as usual   ☐ 1
     I cut down   ☐ 2
     I gave up drinking   ☐ 3
     Never been pregnant   ☐ 4

14. During any of these pregnancies did anyone advise you to stop?
     GP   ☐ 1
     Nurse   ☐ 2
     Midwife   ☐ 3
     Pharmacist   ☐ 4
     Physiotherapist   ☐ 5
     Friends/family   ☐ 6
     Self-help/support group   ☐ 7
     Community group   ☐ 8
     Voluntary group   ☐ 9
     (Specify: _____)

15. If you were to become pregnant in the future, would you:
     Continue as usual   ☐ 1
     Cut down   ☐ 2
     Give up drinking   ☐ 3
     Not relevant   ☐ 4

16. Can you tell me which of the following describes you?
    A person who has taken drugs   ☐ 1
    An ex drug taker   ☐ 2
    A person who has never taken drugs   ☐ 1
                 Go to next section

17. If yes, what drugs have you taken?
    Cannabis   ☐ 1
    Heroin   ☐ 2
    Ecstacy (E.tab)   ☐ 3
    Cocaine   ☐ 4
    LSD   ☐ 5
    Glue sniffing   ☐ 6
    Prescribed drug mixture   ☐ 7
    Valium   ☐ 8
    Other   ☐ 9
    (Specify: _____)

18. Why do you usually take drugs?
    To be sociable   ☐ 1
    To enjoy a night out   ☐ 2
    To relax   ☐ 3
    To cope with depression   ☐ 4
    To cope with family stress   ☐ 5
    To cope with work stress   ☐ 6
    Other   ☐ 7
    (Specify: _____)
    Don't know   ☐ 8

19. If you were ever pregnant, did you take drugs during the pregnancy?
    Yes as usual   ☐ 1
    I cut down   ☐ 2
    I gave up drugs   ☐ 3
    Never been pregnant   ☐ 4

20. During any of these pregnancies did anyone advise you to stop?
    GP   ☐ 1
    Nurse   ☐ 2
    Midwife   ☐ 3
    Pharmacist   ☐ 4
    Physiotherapist   ☐ 5
    Friends/family   ☐ 6
    Self-help/support group   ☐ 7
    Community group   ☐ 8
    Voluntary group   ☐ 9
    (Specify: _____)

Mental health

1. Have you ever felt symptoms of anxiety, depression or stress

	Depression	Anxiety	Stress
Yes	☐ 1	☐ 2	☐ 3
No	☐ 1	☐ 2	☐ 3
Never	☐ 1	☐ 2	☐ 3

2. Have you ever been on tranquillizers/anti-depressants/sleeping pills to help you to cope with anxiety, depression, or stress?

Tranquillizers	Yes	☐ 1	No	☐ 2
Anti-depressants	Yes	☐ 1	No	☐ 2
Sleeping pills	Yes	☐ 1	No	☐ 2
Prozac	Yes	☐ 1	No	☐ 2
Valium	Yes	☐ 1	No	☐ 2

3. If yes, how long were you on them?

Less than 1 month	☐ 1
1–2 months	☐ 2
2–6 months	☐ 3
1 year	☐ 4
Years (State number)	☐ 5 _____

4. What was the particular cause of the stress at the time?

Marital/partner problems	☐ 1
Problems with children	☐ 2
Money problems	☐ 3
Work problems	☐ 4
Bereavement	☐ 5
Inability to cope with life	☐ 6
Loneliness/isolation	☐ 7
Long-term illness	☐ 8
Disability	☐ 9
Health problems	☐ 10
Political situation 'troubles'	☐ 11
Other	☐ 12

(Specify: _____)

5. What do you consider to be the most stressful event in your life?

_____

6. How did you cope with this stressful event?

_____

7.   What else would you normally do to reduce stress?

Talk to friends	☐	1
Talk to family/partner	☐	2
Self-help/support group	☐	3
Spending spree	☐	4
Holiday	☐	5
Eat more	☐	6
Drink more alcohol	☐	7
Praying	☐	8
Talk to GP	☐	9
Talk to priest	☐	10
Talk to nurse	☐	11
Take tranquillizers etc	☐	12
Community group	☐	13
Voluntary group	☐	14
Samaritans	☐	15
Other	☐	16

(Specify: _____)

8.   Have you ever needed treatment from a psychiatrist?

Yes	☐	1
No	☐	2
In-patient	☐	1
Outpatient	☐	2

9.   If yes, have you ever been treated for:

Schizophrenia	☐	1
Alzheimer's Disease (Dementia)	☐	2
Agoraphobia	☐	3
Severe depression	☐	4
Drug related problems	☐	5
Alcohol related problems	☐	6
Postnatal depression	☐	7
Other	☐	8

(Specify: _____)

10. Who has given you the most support through your illness?

Partner/husband	☐	1
Family/friends	☐	2
GP	☐	3
Nurse	☐	4
Community psychiatric nurse	☐	5
Psychiatrist	☐	6
Health visitor	☐	7
Self-help/support group	☐	8

Voluntary agency	☐ 9
Community group	☐ 10
Social worker	☐ 11
Priest	☐ 12
Midwife	☐ 13
Other	☐ 14
(Specify: _____)	

APPENDIX 2

Semi-structured interview questions within a focus group format

1 *Community composition*
How long have you lived here?
Do you know your neighbours?
Do you have friends or relatives in this area that you see often?

2 *Socio-economic environment*
Financial situation
Particular difficulties?
Employment
Housing
Literacy
Education

3 *Community organization and structure*
Organizations of groups
Community activities

4 *Community capacity*
Local leaders
Sense of identity
Part of community

5 *Physical environment*
Conditions
Problems
Transport
Neighbourhood
Environment

6 *Disease and disability profile*
Health problems

Changes
Problems – drugs, alcohol, abuse etc.
Physical disabilities
Learning disabilities

7   *Educational Services*
Locally
Improve

8   *Health services*
Medical services
Access to
Strengths/weaknesses
Suggestions
Hospital services
Access to

9   *Social services*
In use
Positive
Improvements

10   *Miscellaneous*

FURTHER READING

Annett, H. and Rifkin, S. (1988) *Improving Urban Health*. WHO: Geneva.

Blaxter, M. (1990) *Health and Lifestyle Survey*. London: Routledge.

Bowling, A. (1997) *Research Methods in Investigating Health and Health Services*. Buckingham: Open University Press.

Caplan, R. (1993) The importance of social theory for health promotion. *Health Promotion International*, 8(2): 147–156.

Cohen, S. and Syme, S.L. (1985) *Social Support and Health*. London: Academic Press.

Dale, A. and Marsh, M. (1993) *The 1991 Census Users Guide*. London: HMSO.

Department of Health and Social Services (1996) *Health and Wellbeing into the Next Millennium – A Regional Strategy for Health and Social Wellbeing in Northern Ireland 1997–2002*. London: HMSO.

Doyal, L. and Gough, I. (1992) *A Theory of Human Need*. Basingstoke: Macmillan.

Gillam, S., Pampling, D., McClenahan, J. and Harris, J. (1994) *Community Orientated Primary Care*. London: Kings Fund.

Graham, H. (1988) Women and smoking in the United Kingdom: implications for health promotion. *Health Promotion*, 3(4): 371–382.

Graham, H. (1993) *Hardship and Health in Women's Lives*. London: Harvester Wheatsheaf.

Harris, R., Jefferson, C. and Spence, J. (1990) *The Northern Ireland Economy*. London: Longman.

Lazenbatt, A. (2000) Tackling inequalities in health in Northern Ireland. *Community Practitioner*, 73(2): 481–483.

Lazenbatt, A. and Hunter, P. (2000) 'An evaluation of a drop-in centre for working women'. Queen's University of Belfast/Royal College of Nursing, Northern Ireland.

Lazenbatt, A. and Orr, J. (2001) Evaluation and effectiveness in practice. *International Journal of Nursing Practice*, 7(6) (in press).

Lazenbatt, A., McWhirter, L., Bradley, M. and Orr, J. (1999) The role of nursing partnership interventions in improving the health of disadvantaged women. *Journal of Advanced Nursing*, 30(6): 1280–1288.

Lazenbatt, A., McWhirter, L., Bradley, M. and Orr, J. (2000a) Community Nursing Achievements in targeting health and social need. *Nursing Times Research*, 5(3): 178–192.

Lazenbatt, A., McWhirter, L., Bradley, M., Orr, J. and Chambers, M. (2000b) Tackling inequalities in health and social wellbeing – evidence of 'good practice' by nurses, midwives and health visitors. *International Journal of Nursing Practice*, 6(2) April: 76–88.

Lazenbatt, A., Lynch, U. and O'Neill, E. (2001) Revealing the hidden 'troubles' in Northern Ireland: the role of Participatory Rapid Appraisal. *Health Education Research* (in press).

Leventhal, M. (1993) *An Introductory Guide To The 1991 Census*. London: HMSO.

North and West Belfast Health and Social Services Trust (1997) *Summary Report of Issues Raised at Public Health Workshops*. N&WBelHSST Report: Belfast.

Ong, Bie Nio Ong *et al.* (1991) 'Rapid Participatory Appraisal in an urban setting'. *Social Science and Medicine*, 32(8): 14–20.

Oppenheim, C. and Harker, L.(1996) *Poverty: the Facts*, revised and updated version. London: Poverty Action Group.

Patton, M.Q. (1990) *Qualitative Evaluation and Research Methods*. London: Sage.

Poulton, B. (1996) *Multidisciplinary Audit in Primary Health Care*. London: Royal College of Nursing.

Pugh, H. and Moser, K. (1990) Measuring women's mortality differences. In H. Roberts (ed.) *Women's Health Counts*. London: Routledge.

Save the Children Fund (1994) *Poverty is a War Against Children, Who's Poor and Who's at Risk in Northern Ireland*. London: Save the Children Fund.

Scrimshaw, S. and Hutardo, E. (1988) *Rapid Assessment Procedures*. Toyko: United Nations University.

Shamian, J. and Kupe, S.S. (1993) *Community Participation, Primary Health Care and the Nurse in Botswana*. Toronto, Canada: University of Toronto.

SPSS (PC) (1995) *SPSSX – User's Guide*, third edition. Chicago: SPSS Marketing Department.

Taylor, S.J. and Bogdan, R. (1984) *Introduction to Qualitative Research Methods*. New York: Wiley.

Thies, J. and Grady, H. (1991) *Participatory Rapid Participatory Appraisal For Community Development*. London: Save the Children Fund.

Townsend, P., Philimore, P. and Beattie, A. (1988) *Health and Deprivation: Inequality in the North*. London: Croom-Helm.

Varkevisser, C.M. and Alihonou, E. (1993) *Rapid Participatory Appraisal of Health and Nutrition in a Primary Health Care Project in Pahou*. Amsterdam: Royal Tropical Institute.

Wilkinson, R. (1996) *Unhealthy Societies: The Afflictions of Inequality*. London: Routledge.

World Health Organization (1978) *Primary Health Care: Report of the International Conference on Primary Care*. Alma Ata Geneva: WHO.

CHAPTER 11

EVALUATION IN PRACTICE: STRUCTURE

Structure refers to the setting in which the intervention takes place and the resources that are available. It is the easiest of all the phases of evaluation and yet is overlooked in some evaluation procedures. The structure and planning phase of evaluation sets out how you get from a starting point to the end point and what you want to achieve. Some structural aspects of interventions and programmes that can be evaluated are:

- Facilities: accessibility of support services, safety measures, convenience for clients etc
- Equipment: staff ability to use equipment, adequate supplies etc.
- Staff: experience, staff-client ratio, qualifications etc.
- Finances: salaries, funding sources etc.

SETTING UP A DROP-IN CENTRE FOR PROSTITUTES: A WOMAN-CENTRED MULTI-AGENCY APPROACH

Background

Primary healthcare teams are increasingly using needs assessment as a means of developing well-focused care programmes among their practice populations. However, there is often a danger that this process will omit groups of people who are difficult to identify in a population such as travellers, the homeless community, refugees, minority groups including gay men, prostitutes, bisexuals, lesbians, substance abusers, sex workers or even adolescents. The desire to improve the health and wellbeing of such groups may not be the only motivating factor as there are likely to be knock-on gains. For instance, the provision of medical care to a group of local drug users may reduce crime and social stress in the neighbourhood, benefiting the community as a consequence.

Within society there are marginalized groups of people who require health and social care but do not access services such as health checks, screening, well-focused care, self-help or support groups and do not avail themselves of their GP to ask for assistance (see Chapter 2). The problem can be particularly detrimental to the health and wellbeing of prostitutes who may not seek healthcare for several reasons because they may:

- not be registered with any practice
- not know what is on offer because literacy difficulties prevent them from doing so
- feel alienated by the medical establishment
- have a medical fear
- have a concern for confidentiality
- have a language difficulty
- find the services threatening.

The lessons gained from such work have relevance across the whole spectrum of healthcare provision and purchasing. The results can be rewarding not only for the target group, but also for the public health as a whole. By enhancing the health of those in greatest need, standards of healthcare are likely to be enhanced and inequities and inequalities in health reduced.

Rationale for the study

Prostitution per se is not a crime, but it is a crime to solicit publicly. Prostitution is a serious women's health issue as well as a human rights issue and nurses are starting to look at the decriminalization debate (Casey, 1995). Women engaged in this form of employment are subject to abuse and violence from clients, pimps and domestic violence as well as feeling isolated and vulnerable within society. Furthermore, they can be imprisoned for non-payment of fines and their children can be taken into care while they are serving a prison sentence or they can be perceived as 'not good enough' mothers. Since the advent of HIV/AIDS, much research into female prostitution has been undertaken from an essentially behavioural and epidemiological perspective (Whittaker and Hart, 1996).

Indeed, there is substantial evidence that behaviour may influence health status. About 50% of premature deaths in Western countries can be attributable to lifestyle (Hamburg, 1992). Four behaviours have been associated with disease, namely smoking, alcohol misuse, poor nutrition and low levels of exercise – the so-called 'holy four' (McQueen, 1987). More recently high-risk sexual activity has been added to the list. Much of the recent and more systematic research on the health status of prostitutes has either been prompted by or mediated by the moral panic surrounding AIDs, dating from the mid-1980s. Its focus has tended to be epidemiological with emphasis on charting the prevalence of HIV infection. The picture that has emerged is less alarming than many would have predicted. A multicentre cross-sectional survey of women sex workers across nine European societies reported an overall prevalence of 1.5% in non-intravenous drug users and 31.8% in intravenous drug users (European Working Group on HIV Infection in Female Prostitutes, 1993).

In a large London series, Ward et al. (1993) reported an overall prevalence for HIV of 1.7%, and infection in these women was related to either injecting drug use or to sex with a non-paying partner known to have HIV. Not all estimates are as low as these figures in London suggest and there is in fact considerable variation. For example in Glasgow in 1991 it was found that 2.5% of prostitutes were infected with HIV (McKeganey et al., 1992) and in Edinburgh in 1988, 14% were reported to be infected with HIV (Morgan Thomas et al., 1992). The higher percentage in Edinburgh may reflect the inclusion of male sex workers in the sample.

Risk and risk behaviour have become key words in the development of AIDS research (Grover, 1988; McCormack, 1997) and of all the risk factors relevant to determining the distribution of HIV disease, risk behaviour is the most important. HIV is very much a behavioural disease and is subject to variations in the way humans interact and behave. This is particularly pertinent within the relationship between client and sex worker with respect to condom use and drug misuse. Many prostitutes are risk takers and are described as young, inexperienced, in need of money, living in poverty, working on the streets and coming from abusive and violent backgrounds (Barnard, 1993; Faugier and Cranfield, 1995; Bloor, 1995; Plumridge, 1996; Naden et al., 1998). In some studies workers not clients appear responsible for condom use (Browne, 1995; McKeganey and Barnard, 1997; Cusick, 1998). However, Faugier and Cranfield's study of the Manchester sex industry suggests that all workers were keen on condom use with clients but they were less optimistic about the women controlling the situation to their advantage. Moreover, Bloor (1995) has argued that in the developing world, unsafe commercial sex 'is in response to the wishes of the clients, not prostitutes and reflects the clients' domination of the encounter'; in the developed world then unsafe commercial sex 'takes place despite the wishes of the women'. This scenario is particularly important not only for the health and wellbeing of the individual prostitute but also for the population at large.

This pilot project aimed to extend the limited body of knowledge by exploring the occupational health risks which women themselves face when they work as prostitutes in an inner city area (Day, 1990; Scambler et al., 1990; Kinnell, 1993; Faugier, 1996; Lazenbatt et al., 1999b; Lazenbatt and Hunter, 2000;). It explored the wider context of these working women's lives and how this related to their health and safety at work as well as their specific health, social and sexual needs. It pays attention to the inter-related social and sexual inequalities such as violence and sexuality that may impinge on the health of women working on the streets and the problems of access to healthcare services for these marginalized women. The risk of injury and abuse resulting from client assault is known to be high, particularly among street workers. It has been suggested that prostitution 'is very often about violence' as well as sex (Kinnell, 1993; Parker, 1998). One example of similar work is Barnard's research which describes and analyses the conditions of work for street-working prostitutes. It shows how the organization of sex work in Glasgow's red-light district exposes women to various forms of health risk, in particular that of male client violence (Barnard, 1993).

Perhaps the most neglected of prostitutes' health needs are those general needs that are representative of women living in poverty (McLeod, 1982; Farley and Barkan, 1998) as well as the unpredictable, stigmatizing and frequently stressful nature of prostitution. Both relative poverty and threatening life events are known to underlie poor general health status (Payne, 1991; Scambler and Scambler, 1995). Women who prostitute simply do not have the same access to healthcare as others and there is some evidence to suggest that they do not register with GPs (Gallaher et al., 1989). A woman may be nervous about disclosing her profession to a healthcare professional because of stigmatization and the risk of losing her children. Indeed, this reticence about disclosing their work may be understandable in the light of one national study's findings which showed that 36% of GPs approved of HIV testing for women street-workers without consent, and 75% stated that they were willing to share a positive result with practice partners, also without consent (Gallaher *et al.*,1989). This reluctance to confide in GPs and family planning clinics has heralded the promotion of 'outreach' programmes such as the Praed Street Project at St Mary's Hospital in London. These centres recognize that neither the general needs nor the special health needs of prostitutes are being satisfied by the often user-unfriendly routine 'passive' primary or secondary services. The need for treatment, care, advice and support is not always translated into provision.

Pilot project

This project was designed to illustrate the structure phase of an evaluation (see Chapter 7, Stages 1, 2 and 3). The main emphasis of the pilot project was the introduction of a drop-in centre for this marginalized group of women working on the streets and included an assessment of need and an evaluation of the success and efficacy of this outreach programme. The suggested location was in a central city area that served the target population of street-working women within a disadvantaged area. The project management team included members of staff from the Royal College of Nursing (RCN) and a group of university researchers. The project team employed two nurse practitioners on a part-time basis. Both practitioners have a dual role, one as a provider of the drop-in service (nursing care, informational needs, counselling and support) as well as an evaluator of the service (Lazenbatt *et al.*, 1999b; Lazenbatt and Hunter, 2000; Lazenbatt and Orr, 2001).

Aims and objectives

The aim was to provide an 'outreach' drop-in centre for women working as street prostitutes. The nurse practitioners work in partnership with agencies to provide a range of services and interventions that are acceptable and accessible to women and young girls who work as prostitutes in the inner city area.
    The objectives were to:

* establish and maintain close contact with women of all ages who work as street prostitutes in the area
* identify the health and social needs of this marginalized group
* provide an equitable and accessible street-based outreach service, initially two nights per week, to vulnerable girls and women
* provide advice, support and information on a variety of health topics such as sexual health, mental and psychological health and social and physical wellbeing
* provide services such as counselling, self-help and support groups and skills in assertiveness and empowerment
* empower and enable these women to make positive informed choices to aid their health and wellbeing
* assist the women in using existing services.

Partnership and inter-agency working

The structure and planning of the intervention included the establishment of clear channels of communication and agreed practice guidelines with representatives from all agencies likely to have an interest in providing support and advice to prostitutes. Included are agencies such as Barnardo's, Brooke Advisory Clinic, Family Planning Association, Housing Executive, Simon Community, health centres, Salvation Army, GUM Clinics, Alcoholics Anonymous, NEXUS, police, Rape Crisis Centre, Women's Aid etc. Consulting with the wider primary care team in the area was very informative as GPs, pharmacists, health visitors, midwives and social workers knew much about the target population.

Networking with other key agencies provides a closely organized directory of services to address material, economic, social and emotional needs, as well as encouraging self-help and peer group empowerment (see Chapter 7, Stage 2). Preliminary work already undertaken suggests that the main areas of commonality between the agencies and the women with a view to developing a multi-agency initiative are:

- concerns for the women's health including social and mental wellbeing
- the welfare and safety of the sex workers lives
- concerns for the often vulnerable young woman entering prostitution
- options for those wishing to exit prostitution.

The drop-in centre

Accessibility and facilities

As stated, the proposed centre was situated in a commercial district near a major city centre and was accessible and convenient for all women working on the streets. This area covers a square mile and is well known as the city's red-light district. The drop-in service provided a safe environment for the provision of free condoms and an extensive range of information and support services concerning holistic health and social issues such as:

- contraception and provision of condom and prophylactics to cover all sexual services and user groups
- pregnancy and pregnancy testing
- cytology testing
- breast examination
- HIV/AIDS information and testing
- sexually transmitted diseases
- genitourinary problems
- drug abuse
- alcohol abuse
- violence and abuse
- rape
- backpain
- dermatology problems
- sexual health and soft tissue damage

- referral for counselling (abortion, termination)
- mental health issues
- other health problems such as chiropody, dental etc.
- housing problems
- support through individual and group counselling
- social isolation
- problems with violence
- family disruptions
- welfare and legal services
- advocacy for prostitutes
- access to other services.

Safety issues

Preliminary meetings took place with the local police to seek their advice with respect to the safety of the drop-in centre, the nurse practitioners and the 'clients' in attendance. The police were aware of the service, its opening times and suggested that the drop-in centre should have a personal alarm system fitted. The management team also considered providing the nurse practitioners with special training in personal protection and evidence was gathered with respect to its benefits. To increase their safety the two nurse practitioners carry mobile phones so that they can contact help at all times.

Nurse practitioners' qualifications, experience and training

The education of nurse practitioners takes into account basic primary care categories such as internal medicine, paediatrics, obstetrics and geriatrics. These nurses are specialists, with medical and nursing knowledge and skills, that are both combined in a nursing role. They are educated to perform a broad range of primary care interventions that will be required for the delivery of the drop-in centre such as:

- health assessment
- diagnosis
- health education and promotion
- referrals
- prescribing of some drugs
- management of minor illnesses.

Equipment

The drop-in centre requires certain specialized pieces of equipment such as:

- laptop computer
- CCTV
- medical diagnostic equipment such as stethoscope, ophthalmoscope etc
- smear and pregnancy testing equipment

- secure fridge to store blood samples
- secure safe for syringes and needles
- blood testing equipment
- patient's examining couch
- blankets, paper towels etc
- toiletries
- screen
- 5 mobile phones.

Evaluation methodology

Evaluation can analyse a project's structure, activities, and organization and examine its political and social environment. The structure of an evaluation is also determined by the involvement of agencies working in partnership with the target group. This example of an action evaluation of an outreach service for prostitutes sees the practitioner not only as a service provider but also as an evaluator. One major difficulty is that adequate assessment of a service must not itself compromise the effectiveness of that service. If the process of data collection interferes with the efficiency of the service being assessed then that service will not be as effective as it would otherwise have been. However, a service may also be adversely affected by the intrusion of external evaluators. It is tempting to believe that the objectivity of any evaluation depends upon the disinterest of the evaluator but this is not so. Objectivity depends upon the methods employed for data collection and analysis. The valid assessment of any service is therefore not dependent upon external evaluators but upon sound methodology (see Chapter 8, Stages 4, 5 and 6). This is fortunate since it would seem that for most services, economic reality dictates that evaluation and assessment are undertaken by the providers themselves.

The nurse practitioners were therefore trained in evaluation methods and worked with members of the project team to help them define quality criteria based on the client's views of the service gathered from focus group interviews (see Chapter 7, Stage 2). This allowed the practitioner, through the evaluation structure and process, to collect life stories, vignettes and similar kinds of personal testimony about the health and social needs of the prostitutes. In this way the practitioner allowed the women sufficient time to provide fuller, richer and more complex pictures of the ways in which prostitutes think about their health and lifestyle. This was a crucial way of making the evaluation process less of an imposition and more of a shared exploration of issues and a search for action. It also allowed a transparency of process in that women could be given an explanation of how the data would be collected, where this information would go, who would see it and how it would be used. This was also another way of helping the women to become partners in the process (Lazenbatt *et al.*, 1999b; Lazenbatt and Hunter, 2000).

Ethical issues

Sensitive and extremely personal data were being collected from these women and it was therefore important that no value judgments were made about the character of the individual. The primary social and moral obligation was to treat the data with utmost confidentiality and the prostitutes were made aware that any information that was being collected would be protected so that other members of the chain such as pimps would not know the reality of the behaviour of the women and their real life stories. Confidentiality was vital as the women working together would meet each other on the streets and any disclosure could seriously damage the relationship between the women and the nurse practitioner and militate against future potential recruitment. To overcome these problems the women were given an identification number and no names were exchanged or kept on record.

Measures

Traditionally, the evaluation of medical treatments and services has used measures of morbidity and mortality based on clinical and laboratory tests as outcomes. There is now an increasing emphasis on client-assessed outcome measures in the evaluation of care (Jenkins, 1992). This change in emphasis reflects a broader more holistic view of health to include aspects of an individual's physical, psychological and social wellbeing. In order to measure these broader aspects of health, a range of measures have been developed which aim to explore the client's perception of health status and 'quality of life' (see Chapter 8, Stage 5).

The term 'quality of life' is difficult to define and is often used interchangeably with terms such as 'health-related quality of life' and 'subjective health status'. Such interchangeability of terms suggests a lack of conceptual definition of 'quality of life' and most evaluators agree that as it is a multi-dimentional construct, there are a variety of ways to measure it. It is a concept that measures social, mental, emotional and physical health. A number of generic health status profiles have been developed and these assess a range of subjective health status dimensions with different types of clients and patients. One example of these measures is the Short Form 36 (Ware, 1993; Ware and Sherbourne, 1992). This measure is the result of two large studies, the Health Insurance Experiment (HIE) and the Medical Outcomes Study (MOS).

The Short Form 36 (SF-36) contains one multi-item scale measuring eight dimensions of 'quality of life':

1   Physical health
2   Role limitations due to physical health problems
3   Bodily pain
4   Social functioning
5   General mental and psychological health
6   Role limitations due to emotional problems
7   Vitality and
8   General health perceptions.

Scores for each dimension of the SF-36 are calculated by summing across items in the same scale and then transforming the raw scores on a 0–100 scale (0 for poor health and 100 for good health). In addition, the project also uses a standardized measure of psychological health and wellbeing by using the General Health Questionnaire (GHQ). The GHQ has been used frequently in primary care settings and was developed by Goldberg (1972) as a way of assisting GPs in measuring 'psychological wellbeing' among patients consulting them. It is composed of a series of simple questions about changes in a client's life over the previous few weeks and completing it takes only a few minutes. A mean GHQ score in a population or sub-group can be seen as a measure of population morale or overall psychological health.

The data obtained will be used as baseline measures to study the relationship over time between psychological health and other health-related behaviours such as sexual health, alcohol and drug abuse. Although the nature of the service was informal every attempt was made by the staff to take a full medical history and demographic characteristics of the women. As stated this was achieved by using the SF-36 (Ware and Sherbourne, 1992; Jenkinson *et al.*, 1993) to assess the prostitute's 'quality of life' as a multi-dimentional measure of subjective health and the GHQ to assess psychological health and wellbeing. The measures were extended to include additional data on:

- risk behaviour
- condom use and contraception use
- sexual abuse
- drug and alcohol misuse
- gynaecological and pregnancy history
- psychological and mental health
- housing conditions
- measures of stress
- coping skills
- the presence of social networks and social integration
- life satisfaction
- self-esteem
- happiness
- physical fitness.

The influence of social health, including social networks as a moderator of health status, is well known. However, there is now strong evidence that good quality social health may usefully form an outcome for programmes in its own right (Hersey, 1984). As definitions of these concepts vary, the present project defines social health within broad domains of sexual satisfaction, work satisfaction, financial security, family support, and position in the social hierarchy. Measuring each domain of quality of life in this way offers areas for development in health promotion and some consensus of definition can be found to compare outcomes across services.

The service was being developed based on a model of self-empowerment which is individualistic in orientation and rooted in 'informed choice' as well as emphasizing the developing nature of a person's ability to control their own lives and health status through personal growth and self-assertiveness. It also follows the 'community empowerment' model which recognizes the lack of cohesion and solidarity within many marginalized groups and highlights the need for equity of choice (see Chapter 8, Stage 6).

Sampling 'hard-to-reach' groups

Evaluation involving 'hidden populations' such as the homeless, travellers and prostitutes raises a number of specific methodological questions usually absent from work involving known populations and less sensitive subjects. Scientific randomized control trials are not applicable and neither are census-based sampling frames to randomly sample this population. Quantitative designs use 'representative' sampling to make inferences about a whole population whereas qualitative sampling are non-generalizable but provide maximum theoretical understanding of a social process (see Chapter 8, Stage 5). Sampling becomes more difficult the more sensitive the topic under investigation, and the less visible the activity the harder it is to sample. Jenkins (1992) suggests three reasons why random sampling would not be applicable with this sample:

• the potential legal and social sanctions deter respondents from cooperation
• an extremely large sample is needed to achieve sufficient data for an accurate estimation of what is a statistically rare event
• the low visibility of this population leads to lack of ease in locating the sample.

Snowball sampling (recruitment of the sample)

Snowball sampling has been selected to enlarge this specific target group as it is a useful technique for increasing the sample size. The technique uses key informants to provide the names of others who may then be approached and interviewed thus building up a sample among hard-to-reach groups. It has been used very successfully in the field of drug abuse, using current drug users as 'privileged access interviewers' (Faugier, 1996) and may be particularly useful with very hard-to-reach groups such as prostitutes (McKeganey and Barnard, 1997). The nurse practitioner is the link person in controlling the sample by:

• finding respondents and starting referral chains
• verifying the eligibility of potential respondents
• engaging respondents as informal research assistants
• pacing and monitoring referral chains and data quality.

The intervention uses non-random snowball sampling in order to gain insight into the health needs and problems of this target prostitute population. Whilst recognizing the personal bias and distortion inherent in snowball sampling it is a price which must be paid to gain an understanding of this 'hidden' population and is the best guarantee of recruitment to increase the validity of the data. One of the most powerful tools of pluralistic evaluation is that it allows the evaluator to elicit true-life stories and personal testimony. This shifts the focus of power and illustrates that subjects are no longer asked to make their answers fit the evaluator's questions.

Using this methodology may reveal risky sexual practices and the urgent need to promote health interventions among prostitutes and their clients. The experience of collecting data as a nurse and as an evaluator meant gaining a greater awareness and understanding of the health risk behaviour and the physical and psychological status of the woman involved. The two nurse practitioners were in a prime position to utilize their clinical knowledge and experience to further enhance the knowledge base into health and social wellbeing with such marginalized populations.

Data collection stages

Stage 1

This involved interviewing all the central agencies as well as talking to the prostitute women themselves to identify their health and social needs and to assess priority areas. This stage began with members of the project team taking an ethnographic approach and immersing themselves with the prostitutes working on the streets. Using an ethnographic approach allowed discussions with the women without the threat of structured interviews and questionnaires. Ethnographic approaches may strengthen the evaluation and allow the target group to participate in the assessment. Ethically it was important to let the women know exactly why they were being questioned and also to assess their needs and possible recruitment for the drop-in centre. By not pushing the 'women' into conversations and getting to know them a more trusting atmosphere could be developed where the women could talk and share conversations. This style of methodology provided for recruitment of prostitutes to the drop-in centre and allowed them to ask about health issues which might be worrying them and to see the practitioner and the service as a source of knowledge, information and support.

Stage 2

This was the on-going survey or monitoring of the women attending the drop-in centre and involves the use of the SF-36 questionnaire and the General Health Questionnaire. Further data were collected about demography, views of the clinic service and basic information about sexual behaviour, drug use and general health and social needs. There were also short informal focus group interviews in the centre with the women who were using the service to provide a lay perception of their health and social needs and for the assessment of client satisfaction (approximately 10–20 minutes).

Support materials   Self-help materials were provided to allow more complex information to be given than leaflets. These provided substantial information and even in some cases a structural approach to change (Kleges, 1987). Every woman was given an individual folder to hold material that the nurse practitioner presented to her covering detailed information on the area requiring advice, treatment or screening. These information sheets contained up-to-date evidenced-based material in a form that was easy to read and allowed for differing educational backgrounds of the clients. Information sheets also provided the nurse practitioners with baseline material on which to assess reductions in 'risk behaviours' such as increased condom use, reduction in smoking, reduction in alcohol and drug misuse and increases in screening procedures such as breast examination, cervical cytology, pregnancy testing and vaginal infections as well as a more social and psychological profile of the individual prostitutes.

It has been stated that HIV and AIDS are the nursing challenges of the future (Anita, 1997). In considering the need for behavioural change with respect to HIV infection, the use of non-directive counselling was included in the programme. The advice and educational aspect covered the modes of transmission and infection of HIV, the consequences of HIV infection, and safer-sex techniques.

Anticipated benefits and outcomes and how they will be measured

Immediate outcomes

This project was designed to illustrate the structure phase of an evaluation. The project team was delighted that the project became a reality in that one-year funding was received to develop the drop-in centre for prostitutes. The drop-in centre opened in May 1999 and is now well established (see Chapter 9, Stage 7).

Intermediate outcomes

The project not only measures the reduction in health risk factors but provides baseline and developmental measures of holistic health and wellbeing. Outcome measures should no longer be measured simply through cognitive and behavioural change but should include social health and subjective feelings of wellbeing and functioning relevant to a number of health domains, including:

Physical health risk   There was increased condom usage, uptake of cervical and breast screening, increased access to existing services such as GP clinic, hospital clinics, decreased drug and alcohol misuse, decreased smoking behaviour. Mainstream services, both statutory and voluntary, were linked with these marginalized groups.

Psychological health   There was evidence of increased self-esteem, individual empowerment, decreased stress and vulnerability. Facilitation of the involvement of the prostitutes in decision-making could affect their lives in a positive fashion.

Social health   Isolation was reduced and support mechanisms and coping strategies increased. There was a new uptake of services from other agencies and organizations with links with advocacy for these marginalized and isolated women.

Health networks   The multi-agency networking will act as a forum whereby representatives from various agencies can begin to improve their services to working women particularly in the light of violence against women and begin to reduce social inequalities.

Longer-term outcomes

These may include a reduction in social and health inequalities not only for the prostitutes themselves but also for society at large by strengthening individuals, families, communities and alliances (see Chapter 9, Stage 7). The centre may also provide a forum whereby societal and policy issues can be raised with the aim of pursuing health gains and equity for this group of vulnerable women in the longer term.

These outcome measures allow a more composite multi-dimentional measurement of 'quality of life' for this group of prostitutes and illustrate a reduced risk for this high-risk population, with no normal access to prevention and protection services. Evaluation is within a pluralistic framework which allows the use of qualitative and quantitative measures. The evaluation report will provide evidence that the nurse practitioners are:

- understanding and raising awareness of prostitutes' health and social needs
- introducing an awareness of prostitutes' health needs into policy and planning processes of statutory and voluntary organizations
- ensuring the provision of service and support specifically for prostitutes.

Regular on-going evaluation as suggested will allow those providing the service to judge how far its aims are being achieved, as well as involving the client in service planning and structure (see Chapter 9, Stages 8 and 9). However, the evaluation of services needs to go beyond outcome measures and user satisfaction questionnaires to contribute towards policy and service development. This necessitates a knowledge about and understanding of clients' lives. The strength of this approach is that one cannot understand the outcome of a service without knowing how it relates to different stakeholders and agencies. To improve health services we need to understand the client's goals, values, choices, desired aims, constraints and to see how the service changes the balance in these.

This example of an evaluation structure argues for the adoption of a broader concept of evaluation that necessitates new partnerships between managers, professionals, and clients in the assessment process as well as inter-agency collaborations and alliances. Changing the concept of evaluation ensures that clients have a voice within services that are an important part of their lives (see Chapter 7, Stage 2). Such evaluation would lay services open to real scrutiny and could serve to provide a regulatory framework for the pursuit of efficiency and economy and be empowering for both nurses and clients. Therefore, in conclusion, rather than users' views about effectiveness and outcome being at odds with those of professionals, a surprising degree of agreement might be found when clients are involved in the evaluation of outcomes of their healthcare (Lazenbatt *et al.*, 1999b; Lazenbatt and Hunter, 2000).

Budgetary details and outline plan

Establishing a primary healthcare drop-in centre for prostitutes in an inner city area required a minimum of two nurse practitioners and it was envisaged that a substantial amount of the budget would be for their salaries (see Chapter 7, Stage 3). As this was essentially a pilot practice development unit, the nurse practitioners themselves were undertaking practice-based evaluation and data were being collected by the nurse practitioners themselves in order to develop their auditing skills.

Budget breakdown

	£
Nurse practitioner salaries (2 part-time pro rata)	
National Insurance	
Superannuation	
Advertising of posts	

Medical and nursing equipment
Safety equipment
Mobile phones
Printing and postage
Electricity
Supervision and educational support
Computing
Evaluation

Success Indicators	Structure

1   APPROACHES/PARTNERSHIPS

Health alliances/inter-agency
The structure and planning of this intervention includes the establishment of clear channels of communication and agreed practice guidelines with representatives from all agencies likely to have an interest in the outreach centre, e.g. Barnardo's, Brooke Advisory Clinic, Family Planning Association, Housing Executive, Simon Community, Health Centres, GUM Clinics, Alcoholics Anonymous, NEXUS, police, Rape Crisis Centre, Women's Aid etc.

Multidisciplinary
Consulting with the wider primary healthcare team is very informative as social workers, GPs, pharmacists, health visitors and midwives in the area know much about the target population. Networking with other key agencies provides a closely organized directory of services to address material, economic, social and emotional needs, as well as encouraging self-help and peer group empowerment.

2   TOOLS (METHODS)

Needs assessment
Primary care teams are increasingly using needs assessment as a means of developing well-focused care programmes among their practice populations. However, there is often a danger that this process will omit groups of people who are difficult to identify such as prostitutes, ethnic minorities, the homeless etc.

Research
Sensitive and extremely personal data can be collected from these women and it is therefore important that no value judgments are made about the character of the individual concerned. The primary social and moral obligation must be that the evaluation data are

treated with the utmost confidentiality and that the prostitutes are made aware that any information that is collected will be protected. They must also be reassured that other members of the chain such as pimps would not know the reality of the behaviour of the women and their real life stories.

Audit/evaluation

This example of an action evaluation of an outreach service for prostitutes sees the practitioner not only as a service provider but also as an evaluator. Traditionally, the evaluation of medical treatments and services uses measures of morbidity and mortality based on clinical and laboratory tests as outcomes. However, there is now an increasing emphasis on client-assessed outcome measures in the evaluation of care. Outcome measures should no longer be measured simply through cognitive and behavioural change but should include social health and subjective feelings of wellbeing and functioning relevant to a number of health domains. There is now strong evidence that good quality social health may usefully form an outcome for programmes in its own right. The evaluation not only measures the reduction in health risk factors but provides developmental measures of positive holistic health.

3   RESOURCES

Support material

Self-help materials are provided to allow more complex information to be given than leaflets. These provide substantial information and even in some cases a structural approach to change. Every woman is given an individual folder to hold material that the nurse practitioners present to her covering detailed information on the area requiring advice, treatment or screening. These information sheets contain up-to-date evidenced-based material in an easy to read form and allow for differing educational backgrounds of the clients.

Setting

The main emphasis of the pilot project is the introduction of a drop-in centre for this marginalized group of women and includes an assessment of need and evaluation of the success and efficacy of this outreach organization for women working in the streets. The suggested location is in an inner city area and serves the target population of street-working women within this disadvantaged area.

Delivery agent

The drop-in service is staffed by two part-time nurse practitioners and provides a safe environment for the provision of free condoms and an extensive range of information and support concerning holistic health and social issues.

Training of the delivery agent

This example of an action evaluation of an innovative project of an outreach service for prostitutes sees the practitioner as the evaluator. The two part-time nurse practitioners are trained in evaluation methods and work with members of the project team to help define quality criteria based on the client's views of the service gathered from focus group interviews. This allows the evaluation process to collect life stories, vignettes and similar kinds of personal testimony and health and social needs from the prostitutes.

4   INDIVIDUAL COMMUNITY

Holistic Health
Traditionally, the evaluation of medical treatment and services uses measures of morbidity and mortality based on clinical and laboratory tests as outcomes. There is now an increasing emphasis on client-assessed outcome measures in the evaluation of care. This change in emphasis reflects a broader more holistic view of health to include aspects of an individual's physical, psychological and social wellbeing. In order to measure these broader aspects of health, a range of measures have been developed which aim to explore the client's perception of health status.

Culture
Within society there are inequitable groups of people who require health and social care but do not access services such as health checks, screening, well-focused care, self-help or support groups and do not avail themselves of their GP to ask for assistance. The problem can be particularly detrimental to the health and wellbeing of prostitutes and the homeless who may not seek health care for many reasons.

Community development
The service and evaluation follows the community empowerment model which recognizes that often there is a lack of cohesion and solidarity within many marginalized groups and highlights the need for equity of choice.

Empowerment
The service is developed upon a model of self-empowerment which is individualistic in orientation and rooted in informed choice. It emphasizes the developing nature of a woman's ability to control her own life and health status through personal growth and self-assertiveness. Networking with other key agencies provides a closely organized directory of services to address material, economic, social and emotional needs, as well as encouraging self-help and peer group empowerment.

FURTHER READING

Barnard, M. (1993) Violence and vulnerability: conditions of work for street working prostitutes. *Sociology of Health and Illness*, 15(5): 683–705.

Bloor, M. (1995) *The Sociology of HIV Transmission*. London: Sage.

Browne, J. (1995) The social meanings behind male sex work. *British Journal of Sociology*, 46(4): 598–622.

Casey, M. (1995) *A Sexual Health Services for Prostitutes in the UK*. London: EUROPAP, St Mary's Hospital.

Cusick, L. (1998) Non-use of condoms by prostitute women. *AIDS Care Psychological and Socio-Medical Aspects of AIDS/HIV*, 10(2): 133–146.

Day, S. (1990) Prostitute women and the ideology of work in London. In D. Felman, (ed.) *Culture and Aids*. New York: Praeger.

European Working Group on HIV Infection in Female Prostitutes (1993) HIV in European female street workers. *AIDS*, 7: 401–408.

Farley, M. and Barkan, H. (1998) Post violence and post traumatic stress disorder. *Women and Health*, 27: 37–49.

Faugier, J. (1996) 'Looking for business: a descriptive study of drug using among female prostitutes and their clients and their health care needs.' Unpublished PhD thesis, Manchester University, Manchester.

Faugier, J. and Cranfield, S. (1995) Reaching male clients of female prostitutes: the challenge of HIV prevention. *AIDS Care*, 7: S21–S32.

Gallagher, M. *et al.*, (1989) *A National Study of HIV Infection, AIDS and General Practice*. Health care research report, report no 36. University of Newcastle-upon-Tyne, Newcastle-upon-Tyne.

Goldgerg, D. (1972) *Detection of Psychiatric Illness by Questionnaire*. Oxford: Oxford University Press.

Grover, J.Z. (1988) AIDS: keywords. In D. Crimp (ed.) *AIDS: Cultural Analysis*. Cambridge, MA: MIT Press.

Hamburg, D.A. (1992) *Health and Behaviour*. Washington DC: National Academy Press.

Hersey, J.C. (1984) Promoting social support: the impact of friends can be a good medicine campaign. *Health Education Quarterly*, 11: 293–311.

Jenkins, C.D. (1992) Assessment of outcomes of health interventions. *Social Science and Medicine*, 35: 367–375.

Jenkinson, C. *et al.*, (1993) Short Form 36 (SF-36) Health Survey Questionnaire: Normative Data for Adults of Working Age. *British Medical Journal*, 1437–1440.

Kinnell, H. (1993) Prostitutes' exposure to rape. Paper presented to the Social Aspects of AIDS Conference, South Bank University, London.

Kleges, R.C. (1987) A Worksite smoking modification competition: potential for public health impact. *American Journal of Public Health*, 76: 198–200.

Lazenbatt, A. (2000) Tackling inequalities in health in Northern Ireland. *Community Practitioner*, 73(2): 481–483.

Lazenbatt, A. and Hunter, P. (2000) 'An evaluation of a drop-in centre for working women,' Queen's University of Belfast/Royal College of Nursing, Northern Ireland.

Lazenbatt, A. and Orr, J. (2001) Evaluation and effectiveness in practice. *International Journal of Nursing Practice*, 7(6) (in press).

Lazenbatt, A., McWhirter, L., Bradley, M. and Orr, J. (1999a) The role of nursing partnership interventions in improving the health of disadvantaged women. *Journal of Advanced Nursing*, 30(6): 1280–1288.

Lazenbatt, A., Sinclair, M., Hunter, P. and Orr, J. (1999b) A Strategy to target the health needs of prostitutes: a research plan to develop the role of the nurse practitioner in the delivery of primary health care. *British Journal of Community Nursing*, 4(4): 44–50.

Lazenbatt, A., McWhirter, L., Bradley, M. and Orr, J. (2000) Community nursing achievements in targeting health and social need. *Nursing Times Research*, 5(3): 178–192.

Lazenbatt, A., McWhirter, L., Bradley, M., Orr, J. and Chambers, M. (2000) Tackling inequalities in health and social wellbeing – evidence of 'good practice' by nurses, midwives and health visitors. *International Journal of Nursing Practice*, 6(2) April: 76–88.

Lazenbatt, A., Lynch, U. and O'Neill, E. (2001) Revealing the hidden 'troubles' in Northern Ireland: the role of Participatory Rapid Appraisal. *Health Education Research* (in press).

McCormack, N.B. (1997) Prostitutes' wellbeing and risk. *Journal of Sex Research*, 34(1): 62–65.

McLeod, E. (1992) *Working Women: Prostitution Now*. London: Croom-Helm.

McKeganey, N. (1992) *AIDS, Drugs and Sexual Risk*. Buckingham: Open University Press.

McKeganey, N. and Barnard, M. (1997) Sex workers on the streets: prostitutes and their clients. *Journal of the British Sociological Association*, 31(2): 353–360.

McKeganey, N., Barnard M., Leyland A., Coote, I. and Follett, E. (1992) Female street working prostitutes and HIV infection in Glasgow. *British Medical Journal*, 305: 801–804.

McQueen, D. (1987) Research into health behaviour. *Health Promotion and Public Health*, 80: 978–983.

Morgan Thomas, R. (1992) HIV and the Sex Industry. In Bury and S. McLachlan (eds). *Working with Women and AIDS*. London: Routledge.

Naden, S.M. *et al.*, (1998) Antecedents to prostitution – childhood victimization. *Journal of Interpersonal Violence*, 13(2): 206–221.

Parker, M. (1998) Sexual networks and the transmission of HIV in London. *Journal of Biosocial Science*, 30(1): 63–83.

Payne, S. (1991) *Women, Health and Poverty*. London: Harvester Wheatsheaf.

Plumridge, E.W. (1996) Patrons of the sex industry: perceptions of risk. *AIDS Care*, 8(4): 405–416.

Scambler, G. and Scambler, A. (1995) Social change and health promotion among women sex workers in London. *Health Promotion International*, 10: 17–24.

Scambler, G. *et al.*, (1990) Women prostitutes in the AIDS era. *Sociology of Health and Illness*, 12: 260–273.

Ward, H., Day, S. and Mezzone, J. (1993) Prostitution and the risk of HIV: female prostitution on London. *British Medical Journal*, 307: 356–358.

Ware, J.E. (1993) SF-36. *Health Survey-Manual and Interpretation Guide*. Boston, MA: Health Institute, New England, Medical Centre.

Ware, J.E. and Sherbourne, C.D. (1992) The MOS 36-Item Short Form Health Survey 1: conceptual framework and item selection. *Medical Care*, 30(6): 473–483.

Whittaker, P. and Hart, S. (1996) Assessing variability in sexual behaviour: understanding the health risk. In P. Aggleton, P. Davies, and G. Hart (eds) *AIDS: Safety, Sexuality and Risk*. London: Taylor and Francis.

CHAPTER 12

EVALUATION IN PRACTICE: PROCESS

Process evaluation refers to the actual activities carried out by the healthcare providers or the service delivered. It includes the examination of both the process of the programmes's development and delivery and its impact on those to whom it is addressed. Components should include: programme planning and the sequence of delivery, participation rates, participant characteristics, levels of community awareness of programmes, and resources employed for programme implementation. There are several ways to collect process data such as observation, interview, questionnaire or audit. Whichever source of data is used, some set of objectives is needed as a standard against which to compare the activities.

PROCESS EVALUATION OF THE PRINCESS ROYAL TRUST CARERS' CENTRE

Background

Although the activity of caring has been carried out for thousands of years the term 'carer' was little used until the late 1970s. A carer is defined as anyone who is helping to look after a partner, relative or friend who because of illness, old age or disability may not be able to manage at home without help. Nearly 7 million people in the UK are carers; in other words, one in seven adults looks after a relative or friend who cannot manage without help because of sickness or disability (Green, 1988). About 3.9 million carers are women, and in the case of caring for sick or physically or mentally disabled children, almost all the main carers are the mothers (Parker, 1985; Anderson, 1997). About 2.9 million are men and these carers have been invisible for some time, their experience ignored or denied because their unpaid caring contradicts gender norms. With respect to children acting as carers, estimates suggest that up to 51,000 are aged 18 or less and most of them are caring for a parent. By providing services and support for people affected by health problems associated with aging, by mental illness, mental handicap and physical and sensory disability, such carers have become the foundation on which care in the community is built.

Moreover, it is estimated that carers save the government £34 billion every year (Carers National Association, 1997). Without the care provided by friends and relatives, many cared-for people would find themselves unable to live within the community and would have to consider the alternative of residential care which is often very costly. In recent years, the term 'community care' has been used by the government to describe both the support provided by the community and its aim of helping people to remain in their own home environment.

For the first time, in law, the needs of carers have been recognized both in their role of caring and in their own right (DHSS, 1995). Community care helps those who are unable to live alone without help to remain in their own homes and lead the life of their choice by receiving help with personal care, social contact and emotional support. In many cases, this work is undertaken solely by carers who provide 'the great bulk of community care' in partnership with multidisciplinary professionals and supported by social service departments, health services, voluntary organizations and private agencies. Community care, then, is largely, but not solely, about the provision of services to disadvantaged people and therefore involves the re-valuing of people whom society has devalued in some way (Wolfensburger and Thomas, 1994) (see Chapter 2).

The advent of community care has brought the needs of carers sharply into focus amongst professionals who come into contact with older people, people who are sick and those who are disabled, and amongst those who provide information and advice. GPs and other health and social care workers, as well as members of voluntary organizations, have a role to play in supporting carers in their task. According to published guidelines, the Community Care Act is about the empowerment of users and carers (DHSS, SSI, 1991, para 6). In achieving this central aim, care management is seen as 'the process of tailoring services to individual needs'. However, the situation is muddled by the lack of conceptual clarity as to what precisely carers' needs might be and how services can respond to them.

The invisibility and marginalization of caring

The ambiguous position that carers occupy in the policy and service arena has been well documented (Twigg, 1990; Twigg and Atkin, 1994), as has the lack of outcome indicators that can be used to assess whether carers' needs have been met (Hoyes, 1994). The tendency to view carers as 'resources' (Twigg and Atkin, 1994) leads to the all-too-easy assumption that the sole purpose of services is to maintain carers in their role. The persistent failure to see carers in other than instrumental terms means that their own needs, as distinct from the needs of the cared-for person, have rarely been recognized and they have tended to remain 'the unrecognized partners in our welfare system' (Myers and MacDonald, 1996). The relative invisibility of carers means that they are often overlooked in the evaluation process and their inclusion is often more by chance than design.

There are of course a range of other potential carer-related outcomes such as: achievement of autonomy; a reasonable quality of life; the ability to choose whether or not to continue caring; fulfilling expectations for the cared-for-person; and an acquisition of empowerment and coping skills. In relation to the involvement of users and carers in service delivery, the early evidence suggests that far from involving and empowering such individuals, they remain marginalized (Myers and MacDonald, 1996).

Therefore, rather than evaluation starting with the hopes and aspirations of carers, the tendency is for it to focus on deficits and difficulties. Whilst it is maintained that a consideration of difficulties must remain central to definitions of need, a more holistic approach is required if evaluations are to be more than problem lists and if solutions are to build upon individuals' strengths and coping strategies, rather than undermining them.

The hidden burden of caring

Carers are entitled to be informed about the services which are available to them. In addition, their needs must be taken into consideration when planning care packages and their voices should be heard in the decision-making process. However, the burden of caring creates problems for carers as they are often elderly or in poor health themselves, and many have great difficulty in coping with the pressures of the caring role. The negative impact of caring has been well documented (Heron, 1998; Graham, 1994; Evason et al., 1993). Heron (1998) has conceptualized the impact of caring into three main areas – stress, limitations and emotional impact. Caring for someone can be exhausting and emotionally stressful and the carer can often feel isolated, unsupported and alone. Limitations refer to the fact that working as a carer is unpaid and brings no status or contract of employment. Indeed, many people give up their paid job or reduce their hours of employment to care for someone. This means that they may miss out on job opportunities and even face the prospect of financial hardship because they have no chance to build up savings to help meet the extra cost of caring. This combined impact of poverty, isolation and stress can lead to a feeling of 'being trapped' for some carers and in extreme cases this can lead to feelings of depression and helplessness (Heron, 1998).

Carers comprise a large and heterogeneous group, poorly characterized by routine census statistics in the UK (Anderson, 1997). Well-structured comprehensive work with carers in local communities is still at a relatively early stage. One result of this is that there have been relatively few publications which provide straightforward guidance and practical advice needed to plan projects at a local level, looking at the potential pitfalls, costs and management, as well as evidence of 'best practice' (Warner, 1999). Although there is limited research into the actual needs of carers, there is now much more general understanding of the implications of care, in terms of the physical 'daily grind' and the emotional burdens shouldered by carers (Olsen, 1997). The needs of carers are usually defined by professional interpreters, rather than elicited directly from the carers themselves. In fact, few studies or evaluations have investigated the contribution and views of unpaid carers. Until recently these have been grossly undervalued, because the focus of concern was on more formal, medical-led treatments and cures (Ong, 1991).

The Princess Royal Trust Carers' Centre

Background to programme

The Princess Royal Trust for Carers' Centres were established on the initiative of Her Royal Highness the Princess Royal, in October 1991. These centres aim to raise awareness of the needs of carers and provide them with the help and support they need, and in the ways they most want. Over the past five years, the Trust has grown, and there are now over 80 centres across the UK. The Trust does not manage the centres directly, but provides the systems, support and common identity to enable them to form a unified national network. Prudential is the principal sponsor and has contributed cash and gifts in kind, as part of the Prudential Carers Initiative. This project evaluates one such Princess Royal Carer Centre. The centre is managed by a coordinator and includes administrative and volunteer staff. The coordinator requires a mixture of skills, from the ability to publicize the service, to organizing and liaising with funders, securing co-operation and referrals from different professionals, while keeping in contact with voluntary and statutory organizations as well as supporting staff and volunteers. The centre also provide a direct listening and advocacy support service and organizes social outings for carers as well as volunteer recruitment and training in the centre.

Mission

The mission of the Princess Royal Carers' Centre is to:

- provide a place where carers will meet and share together in a setting where there is understanding and appreciation of their individual situation
- provide information, advice and support to carers in ways that are sensitive to their needs and wishes
- encourage the development of local services that are sensitive to the needs and wishes of carers
- be a watchdog about carers' services and work collaboratively to bring full attention to carers' needs.

It also aims to raise an awareness of the needs of carers in local areas and to encourage more carers to seek the support that will make their role easier. The precise range of services is determined through local consultation with the carers themselves and includes:

- providing a listening ear and information, either as a drop-in facility or via telephone helplines
- offering personal counselling and support
- assisting in the arrangements for respite care, or practical help in the home
- advocating on behalf of carers with social services and other service providers
- arranging training, social and recreational events for carers
- networking with other relevant voluntary organizations
- peer support through the training and provision of carer consultants
- self advocacy and empowerment through the Carers' Groups Forum.

How carers are involved in the centre is represented diagramatically in Figure 12.1.

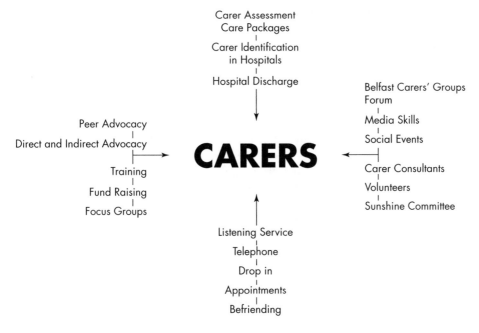

Carer Assessment
Care Packages
|
Carer Identification
in Hospitals
|
Hospital Discharge

Belfast Carers' Groups
Forum
|
Media Skills
|
Social Events

Peer Advocacy
|
Direct and Indirect Advocacy
|
Training
|
Fund Raising
|
Focus Groups

CARERS

Carer Consultants
|
Volunteers
|
Sunshine Committee

Listening Service
|
Telephone
|
Drop in
|
Appointments
|
Befriending

Figure 12.1   How carers are involved at the Princess Royal Trust Carers' Centre

Process evaluation

What is the purpose of process evaluation?

Process evaluation is sometimes referred to as formative evaluation as it is intended to help form the development of a service (see Chapter 5). It generally does not use 'hard' scientific methods and is mostly carried out on services and programmes. The aim of process evaluation is to give people, external or internal to the service, an understanding of how it operates, and *how* it produces what it does, rather than an understanding of *what* it produces within a local setting. It usually deals with:

- inputs (human, financial and material resources)
- activities (baseline information, services, support groups, outreach)
- outputs (consumer/carer satisfaction, referrals to other agencies, volunteer training).

It addresses the extent to which a service progresses towards its objectives and can identify strengths and weaknesses as well as barriers to progress which were not initially anticipated. This information is particularly useful where people want to set up or replicate a similar service elsewhere. Preferred evaluation designs are usually more qualitative and include structured interviews, focus groups and descriptive designs. Importantly, if specific objectives are not being achieved, this information can be fed back to managers of the service with recommendations for change and improvement (see Chapter 8, Stages 4, 5 and 6). This feedback mechanism is central to good project management and should be structured and systematic. Process evaluation, therefore, provides a detailed understanding of how services operate to arrange cost-effective targeting and to inform with clarity and precision those interested in replicating the service.

Data collection

This evaluation of the Princess Royal Trust Carer Centre includes the examination of both the process of the service development and delivery, and its impact on those to whom it is addressed, namely the carer group. Information and data were collected both qualitatively and quantitatively from various components and these are listed below:

- a description of the carers' service including strategic planning targets
- an analysis of the carers' needs, their participation in and outcomes from using the centre
- contextual factors relevant to service operation
- participation rates and participation characteristics
- level of community awareness of the service
- resources employed for service implementation
- an analysis of the benefits to carers' and users' families
- service planning
- an analysis of the services available through the centre
- views of relevant professionals on the centre (sampled)
- an audit of the organizational arrangements of the centre
- a cost-benefit analysis of the centre
- achievement of planned targets and standards
- a sample of carers' voices
- an audit of the impact of the centre on statutory and voluntary bodies.

1 Process as activity

The centre's organizational database

Process as an activity within the centre is seen as service monitoring and takes into account the costs, inputs, activities and outputs. Monitoring allows the coordinator of the centre to track service performance indicators from baseline information to changes over time, to assess whether the service is working to budget, to establish the implementation of planned activities, and produce output measures (see Chapter 7, Stage 3).

Costs   is the carers service working to budget?
Inputs   have financial resources, staff time, premises been committed as planned?
Activities   have planned activities such as new service developments, volunteer training, outreach services been implemented?
Outputs   has an assessment of client satisfaction, empowerment etc. been undertaken?

Monitoring is based on routinely available data gathered at the initial interview with the carer and on information from the feedback questionnaire. The gathering of information is facilitated by the production and efficient operation of appropriate information systems. The centre has set up a sophisticated organizational database to collect information from other agencies and services useful to the caring professions. The database collates baseline data gathered from the Carer Feedback Questionnaires and interviews and provides output information on effectiveness and efficiency (see Table 12.1). It collects data such as:

Table 12.1 Information collated in the database which allows comparisons to be made between baseline measures and changes over time (Dec 1997–Jan 1999)

Condition of person cared for	%	Geographical location of carers	%
Physical illness	22		
Elderly	16	South and east of city	38
Learning disability	13	North and west of city	33
Alzheimer's Disease	10	Not known	27
Mental illness	7	Other	2
Stroke	7		
Severe arthritis	5		
Terminal	4		
Chronically ill	4	*Economic status*	
Sensory	3	Retired	48
Multiple Sclerosis	3	Economically inactive	31
Parkinson's Disease	3	Unemployed	16
Severe respiratory	1	Student	2
Post-operative	1		
Gender of cared-for person		*Relationship to carer*	
Female	62	Mother	19
Male	38	Partner (male)	19
		Father	14
		Other relative	14
		Son	12
		Partner (female)	9
Gender of carer		Daughter	7
Female	58	Sister	3
Male	42	Friend	3
Age of carers		*Assistance given*	
0–15 years	0	Listening	65
16–29 years	4	Information	23
30–44 years	16	Referral	9
45–64 years	21	Advocacy	2
65–74 years	12	Form filling	1
75–84 years	1	Counselling	1
85+ years	0		
Not known	46		
Enquiry subject		*Means of contact*	
Listening	56	Phone-out	31
Benefits	11	Phone-in	28
Aids/adaptions	8	Letter	2
Direct support	6		

Table 12.1 (Continued)

Condition of person cared for	%	Geographical location of carers	%
Respite care	6		
Leisure	5		
Support groups	4		
Education	2		
Training	2		
Befriending	1		
Residential care	1		
Day care	1		
Transport	1		
Housing advice	1		

- area and postcode
- number of carers attending the centre
- provision and use of phone-in and drop-in facilities – e.g. records of days/times available
- employment status, ethnicity and age of carers
- cared-for person – disability/ailment/condition/needs
- details of cared-for person – age, gender, relationship to carer
- outreach sessions – where, when, how many sessions, how many attending
- outreach services – type of services, statistics
- enquiry subject and means of contact
- advocacy on behalf of carers – specific action and results
- recruitment and training of volunteers – numbers and types of training
- involvement of volunteers in the centre and outreach services
- number of volunteers, extent of involvement, services
- assistance given and policy issues
- service referrals, e.g. to other statutory and voluntary agencies, helplines, advice and information centres
- consumer satisfaction survey – details, numbers surveyed, results etc.

Output and feedback from database

Database analysis (see Table 12.1) revealed that most of the carers attending the centre are in the age group 45–64 years. However, the centre appears to have an under-representation of carers who are children under 15 years, or those in the younger age groups of 16–29 years, as well as those from the other end of the age span, the elderly group of 75–85+ years, and from minority groups. The most prominent relationships to the cared-for person were those of a mother or a male partner caring for his wife. The gender mix was female (62%) and male (38%), with women appearing to access the service to a greater extent than men. A large number of the carers were caring for someone with physical illness (22%) and those who were chronically ill (4%). The main reasons for caring were that the cared-for person was elderly (16%) or had a learning disability (13%) or had Alzheimer's disease (10%). The low number of carers accessing the service for information and support for conditions such as stroke (7%), mental illness (7%), for the terminally ill (4%), MS (3%) and Parkinson's disease (3%) suggests that other statutory and voluntary agencies are providing effective support services in these areas or that the availability of information and support should be better publicized.

Most of the contacts were made by telephone with only 18% of the carers actually attending the centre. This is a worryingly low percentage and may be due to the fact that the centre is situated in a busy city centre and people wishing to access its services may have difficulties with travel arrangements and parking. This access problem may be one of the reasons why the elderly group of carers are not attending the centre. Most enquiries are centred around benefits (11%), direct support (6%) and respite care (6%) while 56% wanted a listening ear. The main forms of help and assistance given as a result of contacting the centre were that the carer could speak to someone who listens (65%), they could receive specific information relating to their needs (23%) and they could be referred (9%) to other agencies and organizations.

Working in partnership with other agencies

The centre places emphasis on developing collaborative working with local and city-wide groups and organizations. Most of the coordinator's time is spent developing strategic mechanisms to assist in the provision and quality of locally based services for referrals. Establishing links with other organizations from both the voluntary and statutory sectors is crucial to ensure that carers' needs are being met as effectively as possible (see Chapter 7, Stage 2). The Princess Royal Trust Carer Centre offers a referral scheme whereby the carer can be assured of being referred to an agency which will provide relevant, up-to-date support and information (see Table 12.2). Between January 1998 and January 1999 a significant number of carers were referred to social services 18% (60), or to voluntary organizations such as Citizens Advice Centres 7% (24), Crossroads YC 7% (23), Benefit Helpline 6% (20), and the Carers National Association 6% (19).

Reaching out to carers

Outreach is a vital part of the carers' centre's work, not only because caring responsibilities keep many carers at home, but also because there are many thousands of people who do not realize they are carers. To contact these 'hidden carers' the centre provides mobile exhibition units which visit shopping centres, local women's groups and voluntary organizations to make contact with local communities and assess their needs. To support carers' groups the Carer's Groups Forum (see Forum Membership detailed in Appendix 1) was established and aims to:

- identify and support isolated carer groups throughout the city
- provide these isolated groups with opportunities to network with each other and learn from each other in a peer setting
- offer a voice for carers
- facilitate self-development through access to carers issues at the Princess Royal Trust Carers Centre

Table 12.2 Working in partnership with other agencies: referrals for Jan 1998–Jan 1999

Organization	Referrals	Organization	Referrals
Accept	3	Help the Aged	18
Action Cancer	2	Home from Hospital	3
Age Concern	6	Hospital social worker	1
Al-Anon	1	Housing Rights	2
Alzheimer's Disease	11	Huntington's Chorea	1
Anorexia Society	1	Law Centre NI	11
Arthritis Care	1	ME Association	3
Barnardo's	1	Macmillan Cancer Relief	1
BCH Patient Advocate	1	Maysfield	1
Beginning Experience	2	MENCAP	3
Benefit Helpline	20	Motability	1
British Epilepsy Society	1	MS Society	6
British Legion	1	National Schizophrenia Fellowship	4
Bryson House	5	Newington Carers' Centre	1
Carers Assoc Ireland	1	Rural Carers' Centre	8
Carers National Association	19	NHSS Council	1
CAUSE	6	Association of Mental Health	1
CCMS	1	Housing Executive	4
Citizens Advice	24	Ace Scheme	1
Contact a Family	2	Oaklee Housing Association	1
Crossroads YC	23	Occupational Therapy	2
Disability Action	8	Parkinson's Disease Society	6
Down's Syndrome	3	People Like Us Scheme	2
Dunlewey Substance Abuse	2	PRAXIS	1
Extra Care	2	Red Cross	1
Families in Contact	5	Relate	1
GP	13	RNIB	2
Grange Care	2	Hospitals	2
Headway	3	Samaritans	1
		Social services	60
		Voluntary services	2
Total referrals			333

- identify and endorse the expertise of carers
- offer group training in those areas which are beneficial to group development such as self advocacy and skills and confidence.

To assess their unmet needs, a questionnaire was distributed to the carers in these various groups to discover their views of the services available in the area. The results from the questionnaire are represented in Table 12.3 below.

Output and feedback from the Carers' Groups Forum's needs assessment questionnaire

The results from the needs assessment questionnaire illustrate the differences in unmet needs. Table 12.3 illustrates that over a third of carers (39%) feel that the delivery of respite care and social services assessments requires a lot of improvement. In addition,

Table 12.3 Responses from the Carers' Groups Forum needs questionnaire (n = 54)

Which of the following would you, as a carer, like to see improved?	Needs a lot of improvement (%)	Needs a little improvement (%)	OK (%)	Excellent (%)
Respite care	39	11	10	3
Hospital admissions/discharges	28	21	13	
GP knowledge of carer issues	45	21	13	
Social services assessments	38	14	15	
Carers assessments	45	9	8	
Transport arrangements	28	27	13	3
Domiciliary care provision	27	17	10	
GP training on mental health	42	12	16	
Hospital appointments	23	18	17	

almost half of the group feel that improvements are required for carers' assessments and for the improvement of GPs knowledge of carer issues. Within the area, only 3% felt that respite care and transport arrangements were meeting their needs in an excellent way.

2. Process as progress towards health gain

The most important goal of primary care and voluntary services is to improve the health of carers and users. Health gain can be assessed by linking the inputs, activities and outputs with indicators of user health status such as:

- improved carer satisfaction/knowledge
- changes in carer behaviour, e.g. empowerment, increased self-esteem
- improved uptake of services
- implementation of evidence-based information
- improved partnership and inter-agency working
- efficiency gains and decreased service costs.

These indicators are sometimes difficult to assess as any health gains may follow behavioural change and these may appear some years or even decades later. Also, changes in behaviour are frequently incremental and difficult to ascribe to any one service or programme. Moreover, studies of the effectiveness of formal interventions seeking to support carers and alleviate the burden of caring often examine a diverse range of outcomes and the data do not easily lend themselves to cross-study integration (see Chapter 9, Stage 7).

However, service users are important stakeholders in primary care, whose voices should always be heard. An extensive body of research literature demonstrates that their perspectives differ from those of healthcare professionals (Blaxter, 1995; Nutbeam, 1996). In addition, asking users and carers about their health has been shown to be as valid as clinical measurement in assessments of their health status (Macdonald, 1996). User perspectives can provide an important component of community service evaluation particularly where desirable outcomes cannot be easily defined and there is a need to use indirect measures such as measures of empowerment.

Benzeval *et al.* (1996) stress that empowerment both of communities and individuals should be an important part of policies and services that aim to tackle inequalities in health and reduce social exclusion (see Chapter 8, Stage 4). While there is no specific definition of empowerment or research documenting an increase in empowerment leading to improvements in health, there is a lot of evidence to show that individuals and groups without power experience worse health (Adams, 1996). Whatever way power is measured, all studies cite evidence that social support and ways of coping contribute to health gain in a non-specific, indirect way. With social support subsumed within empowerment, it is conceivable that the psychological state of empowerment may effect health and social status in the same way. Group empowerment offers possibilities for demonstrating direct physical health improvements through group cohesion, and support.

Vulnerable groups such as carers

Loss of power	Feelings/attitudes	Health and social problems
Fear	Powerlessness	
Loss of control	Helplessness	
Desperation	Anger	Leads to illness both social/psychological
Isolation	Anxiety/stress	and physical and reduction in coping
Uncertainty	Low self-esteem	abilities
Weakness	Low self-worth	

Personal development and empowerment through user participation within the carers' centre

Volunteers are an integral part of the functioning of the centre. To participate in the centre they not only need to be recruited, selected, matched and introduced, they also need to be prepared and trained, and above all, supported. They need to be aware of the informational needs of carers and realize that the focus is on the carer rather than on the obvious needs of the cared-for. They also need an understanding of how they can help in developing realistic standards against which to judge the invisible impact of their work. There is evidence to suggest that those who are trained provide a better service (Nutbeam and Wise, 1996). Recruitment of volunteers for the centre is from hospitals, community centres, social services, by word of mouth or by existing carers evolving into volunteers. Training of these volunteers usually takes place every second Monday of the month and sessions have included an induction and orientation of the programme, the development of training needs analysis with and by volunteers, as well as professional presentations from members of staff from the voluntary and statutory sectors. This programme has also included a residential training weekend for volunteers.

A study to measure carer empowerment

A small evaluative study was undertaken to measure empowerment and personal development of those volunteer carers who were participating in the carers' centre (see Chapter 8, Stage 5). Baseline information was collected from five volunteers to assess their self-esteem, self-respect, confidence and coping skills, knowledge, assertiveness and social support networks. This information was gathered from the volunteers using a structured interview format which had both open-ended and pre-coded questions (see Carer Volunteer Feedback Questionnaire in Appendix 2). The interview schedule was divided into three sections, namely, a carer profile, the impact of caring and an evaluation of participation. A qualitative approach was used to allow for a focus on individual feelings and opinions of carers who were experiencing active volunteer participation.

The findings from this small study clearly illustrate that according to the volunteers, active participation had a positive effect on their personal development and feelings of empowerment. Carers reported a growth in self-esteem, confidence, self-direction and assertiveness. Also, for the majority of carers, the experience of participation led to an increased self-awareness and recognition of existing strengths, expertise and coping skills. These findings reflect those of research literature on the benefits of social support through self-help groups (Braye, 1995). Far from being too consumed by their own concerns to want to help others, the findings suggest that carers gain a sense of fulfilment, usefulness and purpose from supporting carers. This in turn can also increase the ability to cope with caring tasks and, as one carer stated:

> After working at the Centre for a morning, you know, getting involved with other issues I come back home to 'L' feeling more refreshed and ready to slip back into my caring role.

This experience of participation was described by the majority of carers as being like teamwork, where decisions were shared, there was mutual support and everyone was valued for their input. However, to involve people, and consult them, is not simply to collectivize them and miss the fundamental problems of individualism and social isolation. Carers are difficult to conceptualize as they see their roles in very different ways. However, the personal development experienced through being involved in the centre was conceptualized by most as a process of personal empowerment. For three carers in the study, participation has been experienced as a journey from powerlessness to a position of more control, in the centre and in life. From an individual perspective, then, the study shows that the practice of participation is intrinsically valuable as a therapeutic tool, through which individuals can be strengthened and gain or regain self-respect, self-direction and confidence. On the basis of feedback provided by the study participants, the following recommendations were made and these suggested that:

- widespread practice among social and health care professionals should focus more on carer/user strengths, expertise and skills
- emphasis should be placed upon fostering a positive relationship and improving channels of commitment between service carer/user and provider
- participation should be flexible and open-ended to allow people to be involved as little or as much as possible

- priority should be given to carers' own accounts and their wants and needs
- further research and evaluation is required to increase the knowledge of the effects of participation on individual and group empowerment
- dissemination of existing good practice regarding carer participation between statutory and voluntary agencies should be increased.

Services such as the carers' centre need to measure the concept of psychological and group empowerment throughout the evaluation process to offer indirect measures of health and social gain and assess changes over time. Within evaluation, empowerment can be both a process and an outcome (Macdonald, 1996; Nutbeam, 1996).

Personal/psychological empowerment – outcome measures

Individual empowerment can be measured by a mixture of concepts such as:

- motivation
- sense of identity
- self efficacy
- self-esteem
- self-confidence
- self-worth
- increasing a person's knowledge
- enabling them to change attitudes and alter behaviour
- acquisition of personal, social and coping skills
- increased competence
- participation
- peer learning/support/mentoring
- gain rights and better access to services
- social support – outside family (statutory and voluntary sector)
            – networks within families and communities

Group empowerment – outcome measures

Cohesive support networks can increase psychological empowerment by:

- using the intrinsic strengths of families and friends, and voluntary and community organizations
- providing social support in groups – expands social networks
- increasing social cohesion
- group participation
- peer learning/support/mentoring
- group problem-solving techniques
- group equity issues

Benefits and outcomes

The findings from this process evaluation cannot be viewed as representative, but it is likely that the inferences drawn can be generalized to carers outside the centre, because caring is such a common experience. The findings may be of relevance to all other agencies involved in commissioning and providing services for carers and their dependants and suggest that process evaluation can examine a number of important questions such as:

- Which aspects of the service are being successfully implemented?
- What factors are facilitating successful implementation?
- Which aspects have not yet been successfully realized?
- What barriers or problems to service delivery have been identified?
- What factors are causing barriers to change?
- Is the service acceptable to different stakeholders such as staff, clients, carers, other agencies?

It is important that any problems or difficulties are identified early enough to allow for necessary modifications to be made before the end of the service or programme (see Chapter 9, Stages 7, 8 and 9).

Immediate outcomes

Successful implementation

- The centre is developing a unique service for carers which has now received national recognition and is enabling 'new' involvement from individuals who were previously isolated and excluded. The partnership and referral aspects of the service have created a structure for participation for carers and their families and provides a mechanism for engagement with statutory agencies and other voluntary organizations.
- The centre shows that carers need to be treated as individuals rather than conceptualized in collective terms. They are carers of other people and their needs are therefore mediated by another person. Carers often see their roles in very different ways and reconciling the individual experience of caring with service planning is seen as more difficult than many predict.
- The service allows on-going structures of consultation with a flexibility to enable interested parties to move in and out of the process. This seems particularly sensitive to the special needs of carers, who may experience peaks and troughs in their caring tasks. The carers' centre is ensuring that the views of carers are used at all times to inform service development and evaluation.
- Carers are specific about the type of informational need and support that would be helpful. They want direct information about their dependants' diagnosis and management plans so that they can reach a decision about their role in the continuing care of their dependant. They also want general information about how to provide care and how to obtain further help and demand more than a simple delivery of information. They want a two-way dialogue with the service coordinator in which their own contribution is valued equally with that of the professional.

- In many cases they want recognition and support for their own roles, not as additional recipients of care, but as peers with professionals in the caring process. They want to be able to influence their dependants' treatment plans as they are formulated and they want professionals to recognize and provide the help that carers themselves need. Although required information is readily available for carers from other healthcare professionals and agencies, the centre is providing an appropriate context for its delivery.

Barriers to implementation

- Early problems of relationships within the centre re boundaries of responsibilities have now been resolved.
- There has been a lack of resources and funding for staff employed directly for the service. The short-term nature of funding and the needs to meet externally imposed targets have also been problematic. The demands of the service have sometimes overtaken the limited number of staff involved in the centre.
- Output from the organizational database suggests that there is a low number of carers accessing the centre for information and support for conditions such as stroke, multiple sclerosis, Parkinson's disease, mental illness and for the terminally ill. These findings suggest either that other statutory and voluntary agencies are providing effective support services in these areas, or that the availability of information and support through the centre should be targeted at these groups.
- Only 18% of the carers contacted the centre using the drop-in facility. This was a worryingly low percentage and may be due to the fact that the centre is situated in a busy city centre and people wishing to access its services may have difficulty with travel arrangements and parking. This access problem may be one of the reasons why the elderly group of carers are not attending the centre. As many carers are elderly or in ill health themselves situating the centre in a more easily accessible position may be more equitable to certain groups of carers.

Intermediate outcomes

Successful implementation

- The promotion of the Carers' Forum is attempting to broaden the range and depth of carer input and strengthening community participation. It allows specific contributions from carers and the promotion of what is important:

  > if more of us were involved in the shaping of social services, it is likely that we would seek to change them to meet the needs of more people
  > (Carer)

- The results from the volunteer survey to measure empowerment showed that personal development experienced through being involved in the centre was conceptualized by most as a process of personal empowerment. For three carers in the study, participation has been experienced as a journey from powerlessness to a position of more control, in the centre and in life. From an individual perspective, then, the study shows that the practice of participation is intrinsically valuable as a therapeutic tool, through which individuals can be strengthened and gain or regain self-respect, self-direction and confidence.

Barriers to implementation

- Assessing the information from the organizational database suggests that the carers' centre has an under-representation of young, elderly and minority group carers. The challenge for planners and evaluators of community care is to move away from a position where services are judged solely by those who are already using them. This serves only to reinforce the exclusion of 'hidden' carers without adequately addressing why they are hidden. Any form of monitoring and planning based on collective representation of existing carers will not address the fundamental problem of these hidden carers. In response to this finding, the centre should arrange meetings and road shows to target children and young adults in schools and colleges of further education, as well as minority groups and elderly people in community settings.
- The centre should now be aware that leaflets aimed at people within supermarkets, who do not necessarily see themselves as carers, are less likely to stimulate participation, than appropriately organized community sessions in schools, colleges, churches, support groups, minority groups etc.
- A major barrier to achieving 'best practice' concerns the resources available to develop services. The identification of needs that cannot be met due to lack of resources results in centre staff becoming disillusioned and having low morale. There has been a number of resource problems within the centre and this has resulted in staff shortages and the inability to open the centre, at certain times, if the required members of staff are absent or ill. This places extra burdens on the coordinator and produces a paradoxical situation, in which she is required simultaneously to expand the centre's role and to ration demand.

Longer-term outcomes

- Recognition of the value of the contribution which carers make to society is increasing but there is a long way to go. The carers' centre has a vision of a society in which carers are properly valued and supported by government and community and thus enabled to share and fulfil their caring role as effectively as possible. Consultation with carers must be part of a strategy of explicit service development. Carers should see the impact of their involvement, and should be fully aware of what is and is not on the agenda with regard to the discretion that government has in the planning process.
- At a regional level, social services, PAMS and medical and nursing schools need to recognize the importance of carers in healthcare delivery and also to educate these professionals and nursing students and doctors to value the contribution that carers can make as an integral part of routine patient care.

Success Indicators	Process Evaluation

1 APPROACHES/PARTNERSHIPS

Health alliances/inter-agency
The centre places emphasis on developing collaborative working with local and city-wide groups and organizations. Most of the coordinator's time is spent developing strategic work to develop the provision and quality of locally based services for referral mechanisms. Establishing links with other organizations from both the voluntary and statutory sectors is crucial to ensure that carers' needs are met as effectively as possible.

Multidisciplinary
Community care helps people who are unable to manage to live alone without help to remain in their own homes and lead the life of their choice by having help with personal care, social contact and emotional support. In many cases, this work is undertaken solely by carers who provide 'the great bulk of community care' in partnership with multidisciplinary professionals and supported by social service departments, health services, voluntary organizations and private agencies.

2 TOOLS (METHODS)

Evaluation
Process evaluation is sometimes referred to as formative evaluation as it is intended to help form the development of a service. It does not use 'hard' scientific methods and is mostly carried out on services and programmes. The aim of process evaluation is to give people external or internal to the service an understanding of how it operates, and how it produces what it does, rather than an understanding of what it produces within a local setting. It addresses the extent to which a service progresses towards its objectives and can identify strengths and weaknesses as well as barriers to progress which were not initially anticipated. This information is particularly useful where people want to set up or replicate a similar service elsewhere.

Research
Preferred evaluation designs are usually more qualitative and include structured interviews, focus groups and descriptive designs. However, services such as the carers' centre need to measure the concept of psychological and group empowerment throughout the evaluation process to offer indirect measures of health and social gain and assess changes over time.

Needs assessment
The persistent failure to see carers in other than instrumental terms means that their own needs, as distinct from the needs of the cared-for person, have rarely been recognized and they have tended to remain 'the unrecognized partners in our welfare system'. The relative invisibility of carers means that they are often overlooked in the evaluation process and their inclusion is often more by chance than design. To contact these 'hidden' carers, the

centre provides mobile exhibition units which visit shopping centres, local women's groups and voluntary organizations to contact with local communities and assess their needs.

3 RESOURCES

Support material
The centre has set-up a sophisticated organizational database to collect information from other agencies and services useful to the centre. The database collates baseline data gathered from the carer feedback questionnaires and interviews and provides output information on effectiveness and efficiency.

Setting
Although required information is readily available for carers from other healthcare professionals the centre is providing an appropriate context for its delivery. However, only 18% of the carers have contacted the centre using the drop-in facility. This is a worryingly low percentage and may be due to the fact that the centre is situated in a busy city-centre and people wishing to access its services may have difficulty with travel arrangements and parking. This access problem may be one of the reasons why the elderly group of carers are not attending the centre.

Delivery agent
The centre is managed by a coordinator, administrative and volunteer staff. The coordinator requires a mixture of skills from publicizing the service, organizing and liaising with funders, securing co-operation and referrals from multi-professionals, while keeping in contact with voluntary and statutory organizations as well as supporting staff and volunteers.

Training delivery agent
Volunteers are an integral part of the functioning of the centre. They require training and need to be aware of information about other help available and procedures for obtaining it and in understanding problems of carers and those they care for. Sometimes they need to realize the focus is on the carer rather than on the obvious needs of those they care for. Volunteers also need help in understanding how they can help in developing realistic standards against which to judge the visible impact of the work.

4 INDIVIDUAL/COMMUNITY

Holistic health
In relation to the involvement of users and carers, the early evidence suggests that far from involving and empowering such individuals, they remain marginalized. Therefore, rather than evaluation starting with the hopes and aspirations of carers, the tendency is for it to focus on deficits and difficulties. Whilst it is maintained that a consideration of difficulties must remain central to definitions of need, a more holistic approach is required if evaluations are to be more than problem lists and if solutions are to build upon individuals' strengths and coping strategies, rather than undermining them.

Culture

Caring for someone can be exhausting and emotionally stressful and the carer can often feel isolated, unsupported and alone. Working as a carer is unpaid and brings no status or contract of employment. Indeed, many people give up their paid job or reduce their hours of employment to care for someone. This means that they may miss out on job opportunities and even face the prospect of financial hardship because they have no chance to build up savings to help meet the extra cost of caring.

Community development

The advent of community care has brought the needs of carers sharply into focus amongst professionals who come into contact with the elderly, the sick and the disabled, and amongst those who provide information and advice. GPs and other health and social care workers, as well as members of voluntary organizations, have a role to play in supporting carers in their task.

Empowerment

Empowerment both of communities and individuals should be an important part of policies and services that aim to tackle inequalities in health and reduce social exclusion. While there is no specific definition of empowerment, nor research documenting an increase in empowerment leading to improvements in health, there is a lot of evidence to show that individuals and groups without power experience worse health. Whatever way power is measured all studies cite evidence that social support and improved ways of coping contribute to health gain in a non-specific, indirect way.

APPENDIX 1

Carers' Groups Forum membership

174 Disability Project
Action for Dysphasic Adults
AIDS Helpline
Alzheimer's Disease Society
West City Carers Group
CAUSE
Chest, Heart and Stroke
Eating Disorders Association
Everton Carers Group
Families in Contact
Headway
Edgecumbe TRC Carers Group
Huntington's Chorea Association

Mount Oriel Carers Group
NSF Carers Group
Newington Carers Group
North City Carers Group
Orchardville Society
PAPA Resource Centre
Parkinson's Disease Society
South City Carers Group
Suffolk Parents and Carers Group
Downs Syndrome Association
Glenluce Carers
Multiple Sclerosis Society

APPENDIX 2

Carer volunteer feedback questionnaire

Part 1: Carer's profile

1. What is your relationship with the person you care for at present?

    Husband ☐   Wife ☐   Mother ☐   Father ☐
    Daughter ☐   Son ☐   Brother ☐   Sister ☐

    Other relative ☐   Neighbour ☐

2. What age group do you, the carer, fall into?

    Under 25 ☐   25–34 ☐   35–54 ☐   55–64 ☐

    65–74 ☐   75 or over ☐

3. What age group does/did the person you care for belong to?

    Under 25 ☐   25–34 ☐   35–54 ☐   55–64 ☐

    65–74 ☐   75 or over ☐

4. Do you look after anyone else?

    Yes ☐   No ☐

    If yes who? _____

    How many people have you cared for in your life so far? _____

5. Do you live in the same house as the person you care for?

    Yes ☐   No ☐

6. How long have you been caring in your present situation?

    > 1 year ☐   1–5 years ☐   6–10 years ☐

    11–15 years ☐   < 15 years ☐

7. How many hours do you spend caring each week?

    > 5 hours ☐   5–15 hours ☐   16–24 hours ☐

    25–35 hours ☐   36–44 hours ☐   45–60 hours ☐

Part 2: Impact of caring

8.   How long after you started looking after this person did you consider yourself to be a carer?

Immediately ☐   Up to 6 months after ☐

7 months to a year ☐   2–3 years ☐

6–10 years after ☐   10 years after ☐

9.   Since becoming a carer do any of the following refer to you?

Loss or gain of status/income

Strongly agree ☐   Agree ☐   Neither ☐   Disagree ☐
Strongly disagree ☐

Loss or gain of expectations (e.g. career, education)

Strongly agree ☐   Agree ☐   Neither ☐   Disagree ☐
Strongly disagree ☐

Loss or gain of feelings of self-esteem

Strongly agree ☐   Agree ☐   Neither ☐   Disagree ☐
Strongly disagree ☐

Loss or gain of specialized skills (e.g. IT skills, teaching)

Strongly agree ☐   Agree ☐   Neither ☐   Disagree ☐
Strongly disagree ☐

10. To what extent has your role as carer restricted any of the following?

A lot/Not so much/Neither

Pursuit of personal interests/hobbies   ☐   ☐   ☐

Pursuit of employment/career opportunities   ☐   ☐   ☐

Socializing

11. To what extent have you experienced the following during caring?

Feelings of:

| Isolation | Frequently | ☐ | Occasionally | ☐ |
| | Almost never | ☐ | Never | ☐ |

| Personal loneliness | Frequently | ☐ | Occasionally | ☐ |
| | Almost never | ☐ | Never | ☐ |

| Feeling trapped | Frequently | ☐ | Occasionally | ☐ |
| | Almost never | ☐ | Never | ☐ |

| Physical exhaustion | Frequently | ☐ | Occasionally | ☐ |
| | Almost never | ☐ | Never | ☐ |

| Mental exhaustion | Frequently | ☐ | Occasionally | ☐ |
| | Almost never | ☐ | Never | ☐ |

| Depression | Frequently | ☐ | Occasionally | ☐ |
| | Almost never | ☐ | Never | ☐ |

| Powerlessness over situation | Frequently | ☐ | Occasionally | ☐ |
| | Almost never | ☐ | Never | ☐ |

| Hopelessness | Frequently | ☐ | Occasionally | ☐ |
| | Almost never | ☐ | Never | ☐ |

12. Prior to becoming involved with the centre did you have someone to talk to about your needs?

Yes ☐   No ☐

Please specify _____

Part 3: Evaluation of service

13. How did you first hear about the Carers' Centre?

Another carer	☐	Friends	☐	Television	☐
Advice agency	☐	GP	☐	Leaflets	☐
Radio	☐	Newspaper	☐		

Other, please specify _____

14. Initially, why did you wish to use this service?

Benefits Advice ☐   Info. about support services ☐

Emotional support ☐   Info. about rights/entitlements ☐

Enlarge social network ☐   Info. about careers centre ☐

Other, please specify _____

15. What motivated you to become more actively involved with the carers' centre?

_____

_____

16. In what ways have you been invited to participate in this service?

Fundraising ☐   Administration ☐

Management discussions ☐   Staff/carer training ☐

Promotion of service ☐   Counselling ☐

Self-help groups ☐   Staff recruitment ☐

Other, please specify _____

17. What sort of training if any were you provided with?

_____

_____

_____

18. Do you feel there is a need for training?

Yes ☐   No ☐

Why? _____

_____

_____

19. Has being involved in the above activities, enabled you to develop as a person?

Yes ☐   No ☐

20. In what ways?

_____

_____

21. To what extent do you agree with the following statements?

'People are encouraged to be involved all the time. The gain of this way of working is that it gives people confidence.'

Strongly agree ☐ Agree ☐ Neither ☐ Disagree ☐
Strongly disagree ☐

'Through being involved I have been given the opportunity to develop my skills in working with other professionals.'

Strongly agree ☐ Agree ☐ Neither ☐ Disagree ☐
Strongly disagree ☐

'The carer centre is a supportive environment where people gain or regain self-esteem and confidence gaining more control over their lives.'

Strongly agree ☐ Agree ☐ Neither ☐ Disagree ☐
Strongly disagree ☐

'It is important to participate so that other people don't make choices for you. It makes you feel good about yourself and helps make sure you get what you want not what other people want for you.'

Strongly agree ☐ Agree ☐ Neither ☐ Disagree ☐
Strongly disagree ☐

22. Refer back to question 11.

23. As a result of participating in the centre what would you say are the advantages?

_____
_____
_____
_____

FURTHER READING

Adams, R. (1996) *Social Work and Empowerment*. London: Macmillan.

Anderson, R. (1997) The unremitting burden on carers. *British Medical Journal*, 294:6564, 73–74.

Blaxter, M. (1997) Whose fault is it : people's own reasons for inequality in health. *Social Science and Medicine*, 44(6): 747–756.

Benzeval, M., Judge, K. and Whitehead, M. (1996) *Tackling Inequalities in Health: An Agenda for Action*. London: Kings Fund.

Braye, S. (1995) *Empowering Practice in Social Care*. Buckingham: Open University Press.

Carers National Association (1997) *Still Battling? The Carers Act One Year On*. London: CNA.

Department of Health and Social Services Inspectorate SSI (1991) *Care Management and Assessment: Practitioners Guide*. HMSO: London.

Department of Health and Social Services (1995) *Where Next for Carers? Findings from the SSI Project*. Wetherby: DoH.

Evason, E., Knowles, L. and Whittington, D. (1993) *The Cost of Caring*. Joint report by EDC (NI), Centre for Social Research: University of Ulster.

Graham, C. (1994) *The Carers Perspective: An Evaluation of the Effectiveness of Quality Support Services for Carers in North Belfast*. London: CNA.

Green, H. (1988) *Informal Carers: A Study Carried out on behalf of the DHSS as part of the 1985 General Household Survey*. London: HMSO.

Haffenden, S. (1991) *Getting it Right for Carers*. London: HMSO.

Heron, D. (1998) *Working with Carers*. London: Jessica Kingsley.

Hoyes, L. (1994) *Community Care in Transition*. York: Joseph Rowntree Foundation.

King's Fund Informal Carers Unit (1981) *Taking a Break: a Guide for People Caring at Home*. London: King's Fund.

Lazenbatt, A. (1997) *Targeting Health and Social Need, Volume 1: The Contribution of Nurses, Midwives and Health Visitors*. Belfast: The Stationery Office.

Lazenbatt, A. (1999) *Manual for Evaluation and Effectiveness in Practice*, Volume 2. Belfast: The Stationery Office.

Lazenbatt, A. (2000) Tackling inequalities in health in Northern Ireland. *Community Practitioner*, 73(2): 481–483.

Lazenbatt, A., McWhirter, L., Bradley, M. and Orr, J. (1999) The role of nursing partnership interventions in improving the health of disadvantaged women. *Journal of Advanced Nursing*, 30(6): 1280–1288.

Lazenbatt, A., McWhirter, L., Bradley, M. and Orr, J. (2000a) Community nursing achievements in targeting health and social need. *Nursing Times Research*, 5(3): 178–192.

Lazenbatt, A., McWhirter, L., Bradley, M., Orr, J. and Chambers, M. (2000b) Tackling inequalities in health and social wellbeing – evidence of 'good practice' by nurses, midwives and health visitors. *International Journal of Nursing Practice*, 6(2) April: 76–88.

Lazenbatt, A., Lynch, U. and O'Neill, E. (2001) Revealing the hidden 'troubles' in Northern Ireland: the role of Participatory Rapid Appraisal. *Health Education Research* (in press).

Macdonald, G. (1996) Where next for evaluation? *Health Promotion International*, 11(3): 326–330.

Myers, F. and MacDonald, C. (1996) Power to the people? Involving users and carers in needs assessment and care planning – views from the practitioner. *Health and Social Care in the Community*, 4(2): 86–95.

Nutbeam, D. (1996) Achieving 'best practice' in health promotion, *Health Education Research*, 11(3): 317–326.

Nutbeam, D. and Wise, M. (1996) Planning for health for all. *Health Promotion International*, 11(3): 219–226.

Olsen, R. (1997) Carers and the missing: changing professional attitudes. *Health and Social Care in the Community*, 5(2): 116–123.

Ong, B.N. (1991) Researching needs in district nursing, *Journal of Advanced Nursing*, 16: 638–47.

Parker, G. (1985) *With Due Care and Attention: A Review of Research on Informal Care*. Occasional paper 2. London: Family Policy Studies.

Stalker, K. (1990) *Share the Care: an Evaluation of a Family-based Respite Service*. London: Jessica Kingsley.

Twigg, J. (1990) Models of carers: how do social care agencies conceptualize their relationship with informal carers? *Journal of Social Policy*, 18: 53–66.

Twigg, J. (1993) *Policy and Practice in Informal Care*. Buckingham: Open University Press.

Twigg, J. and Atkin, K. (1994) *Carers Perceived: Policy and Practice in Informal Care*. Buckingham: Open University Press.

Warner, L. and Wexler, S. (1998) *Eight Hours a Day and Taken for Granted?* London: The Princess Royal Trust for Carers.

Warner, L. (1999) *Seven and a Half Minutes Is Not Enough*. London: The Princess Royal Trust for Carers.

Wolfensburger, W. and Thomas, S. (1994) Obstacles in the professional human service culture to implementation of the social role and the community integration of clients. *Care in Place*, 1: 53–56.

CHAPTER 13

EVALUATION IN PRACTICE: OUTCOME

The following is an example of the most structured kind of evaluation design. The randomized controlled trial or quasi-experimental study has always been popular with 'scientific' research, as it appears to deal with 'hard facts' rather than subjective opinions. It is good for testing theory or for generating theory as it identifies variables for manipulation and measurement. However, it is often criticized as being totally unnatural, as what happens in a laboratory situation is not likely to happen in ordinary life. Often true experiments are impossible even in principle. This breastfeeding study illustrates a quasi-experimental design with pre-and post-intervention groups: one receiving a 'telemedicine link' and the other acting as a 'control'. The groups are naturally occurring and allocation to them is not under the control of the evaluator.

THE EFFECTIVENESS OF TELEMEDICINE AS A SUPPORT SYSTEM TO ENCOURAGE BREASTFEEDING

Background

Breastfeeding is an ideal way of providing food for the health, growth and development of babies and infants. It offers a range of advantages to both mother and baby. For example, breastfed babies are at a lower risk of infection, particularly gastrointestinal, respiratory and urinary tract. It also offers some protection against allergic disease, particularly where there is a family incidence, and reduces the risk of juvenile onset diabetes. Improved intellectual development is also associated with breastfeeding in healthy term infants (Jones, 1986; Rajan, 1993). For low birthweight infants, it is associated with a reduced risk of mortality – necrotizing entercolitis (Foster *et al.*, 1997). Indeed, UNICEF states in the literature that over a million babies die from unsafe bottle feeding every year. For the mother, it is associated with lower rates of pre-menopausal breast cancer and some forms of ovarian cancer. It can also help with weight loss postnatally and offers unique close contact between the mother and her baby.

However, the prevalence of breastfeeding has declined in many parts of the world for a variety of social, economic and cultural reasons. Social class, age, smoking habit and the age at which the mother completed full-time education are all related to the incidence of breastfeeding. Its incidence is higher among women from higher social classes, older first-time mothers, non-smokers and those who have continued education beyond the age of 18 years (Horton, 1996). In addition, birth order influences breastfeeding, with rates highest among first-time mothers. Also, the feeding method chosen for the first child influences how subsequent siblings are fed.

Breastfeeding statistics

The Office for National Statistics (1995) recently published a report of their 1995 UK Infant Feeding Survey, which demonstrates a statistically significant increase in breastfeeding in all UK countries between 1990 and 1995, and a clear, continuing social class gradient in feeding patterns. The geographical gradient continues with the highest initiation rates occurring in London and the south-east and the lowest rates in northern England, Scotland and Northern Ireland. The highest incidence and duration of breastfeeding occurs in women from social class 1, with an initiation rate of 90% falling to 73% at six weeks post delivery. In contrast, in social class 5 the initiation rate is 50% falling to 23% by six weeks (Foster et al., 1997).

In England and Wales it appears that breastfeeding rates increased from an incidence of 64% in 1990 to 68% in 1995. In England, Scotland and Wales the recent increases follow a period since 1980 in which rates have shown little change. However, the greatest increase since 1990 has occurred in Northern Ireland (ONS, 1995; Foster et al., 1997). Rates have increased from 36% in 1990 to 45% in 1995. It must be stressed, however, that this incidence in 1995 was still lower than elsewhere in the UK which suggests that, despite the effort to promote breastfeeding in Northern Ireland, it remains lower than any other NHS region, and is ranked one of the lowest in Europe (DHSS, 1997; Gordon, 1998). In addition, the duration of breastfeeding for those women who choose to do so, is significantly lower within the province, although there has been some improvement between 1990 and 1995 (DHSS, 1997). By six weeks after birth, less than half (49%) of Northern Ireland mothers who had initiated breastfeeding were continuing to do so (White et al., 1992).

Barriers to breastfeeding

Northern Ireland is recognized as a bottle-feeding culture. Many mothers claim that if they had received more consistent advice and support from informed health professionals, they might have breastfed for longer and more successfully (Morgan, 1985; Jones, 1986; Rajan, 1993). Evidence therefore suggests that lack of professional effectiveness has been shown to be one of the first barriers to successful breastfeeding (Cole, 1977; White et al., 1992). Gordon (1998) suggests that it is the historical medicalization of childbirth in Northern Ireland and control of infant nutrition that has resulted in rigid hospital routines and practices. Indeed, voluntary organizations such as the National Childbirth Trust and La Leche have brought to light the neglect of breastfeeding in some hospitals.

It is apparent from research that there are a host of factors that may affect breastfeeding practice. For many women decisions are often made before conception, guided by religious, cultural and social influences, while the attitudes of health professionals may influence breastfeeding both antenatally and postnatally (Oakley and Rajan, 1993; Kendell, 1995). Financial pressures may mean that many women have to work outside the home and, if the workplace is unable to provide facilities for the continuation of breastfeeding, then these women may decide not to start at all or to discontinue before returning to work. Also, free formula samples to new mothers before discharge from hospital have also been shown to reduce the incidence and duration of breastfeeding (Basire, 1997).

In addition, many studies have explored the reasons why women stop breastfeeding and have concluded that there are a variety of factors which may affect this. These include physical factors such as sore and cracked nipples (Jones, 1984; ONS, 1997); perceived insufficient milk supply (Hillervik and Hofvander Sjoln, 1977; Kvist et al., 1996; ONS, 1997); lack of professional and social support (Jones and West, 1986; Richardson and Champion, 1992); limited antenatal education/knowledge (Wiles, 1984; Richardson and Champion, 1992). Hospital policies/midwifery practices (Wylie and Verber, 1994) and psychological factors such as attitudes to breastfeeding may also influence women's decision to discontinue (Wylie and Verber, 1994; Lynch et al., 1986; ONS, 1997). However, there is evidence to suggest that several of these problems might be prevented if health professionals were to show the mothers how to position the baby correctly and to offer higher levels of practical and emotional support to the mother (Inch and Renfrew, 1989; Inch, 1996).

Lack of support with breastfeeding

Although several studies suggest that health professionals have relatively little influence on a woman's decision relating to feeding (Purtell, 1994; Libbus, 1992), the WHO suggests that, unwittingly, health services may have contributed to the decline in breastfeeding by either failing to support and empower mothers to breastfeed or by introducing routines and procedures that interfere with its establishment (WHO/ UNICEF, 1989; Rea et al., 1997). The failure of medical, midwifery and nursing staff to provide sufficient equitable support and encouragement was identified as a major factor militating against successful breastfeeding for mothers (Rajan, 1993; Rea et al., 1997). Approximately 12% of women who commence breastfeeding discontinue by the time they leave hospital (Foster et al., 1997) and although the reasons are varied, the influence of hospital practices and health professionals is particularly important at this time. Many women frequently express disappointment in the support that they are offered by health professionals (Rea et al., 1997).

When mothers are asked to identify the person who provides the most support for their decision to breastfeed, fathers frequently head the list (Voss et al., 1993; Libbus, 1994; Freed, 1994). In addition, fathers assist mothers with breastfeeding and influence its duration (Buckner, 1993). Research studies in which the fathers themselves are subjects have added to our understanding of their attitudes, knowledge, and difficulties regarding breastfeeding. It is interesting to note that findings from a recent ethnographic study of two communities in Northern Ireland suggest that embarrassment and negative attitudes by men are significant deterrents to breastfeeding for materially deprived families (Moore et al., 1997). Indeed, the incidence of gastroenteritis, chest infections, asthma and repeated urinary tract infections – all conditions which are claimed to be less prevalent in breastfed babies – is significantly higher in this social group (see Chapter 2).

Baby-Friendly Status

The UNICEF baby-friendly initiative is a global campaign run jointly with the World Health Organisation (WHO) to raise breastfeeding rates (WHO/UNICEF, 1989). The initiative encourages hospitals to strive towards and achieve ideal quality standards. Attaining Baby-Friendly Status is a significant challenge for many hospitals. Hospitals have to implement a 10-step plan for successful breastfeeding covering everything from staff training to rooming-in, artificial teats and complementary feeding policies. In addition, they should have a success rate of 50% of mothers who are still breastfeeding at time of discharge. Not all mothers may wish to convert to breastfeeding, but those who wish to do so should be empowered and facilitated by midwives. Hospitals that have not yet reached these goals may be awarded a Certificate of Commitment for implementing the 10-step plan within two years. To date, only three hospitals have achieved Baby-Friendly Status; all stress that they provide appropriate support for mothers, but their major challenge is to extend the duration of the women's breastfeeding.

Breastfeeding statistics from the case study maternity hospital described below illustrate that 57% of mothers are being discharged as breastfeeders; however, this figure drops in the community to 38%. Many women abandon breastfeeding when they face difficulties or lack of support at home. Attainment of Baby-Friendly Status requires hospitals to establish breastfeeding support groups to provide assistance to mothers after discharge. The present study assessed the use of a telemedicine link within a maternity hospital as such a support system for mothers. The technology involved was intended to act as a support system or peer network to prolong the duration of breastfeeding in the community. This may in the longer-term assist the maternity hospital in attaining Baby-Friendly Status.

Telemedicine

The use of telemedicine has been reported in a variety of forms, from the 1960s onwards, and it has been defined in a variety of ways, for example Scannell et al. (1995) provide a very broad definition:

> Telemedicine is the telecommunication of medical diagnosis and patient care. It involves the use of technology as a medium for the provision of medical services to sites that are at a distance from the provider. The concept encompasses everything from the use of standard telephone service through high speed, wide-band width transmission of sophisticated peripheral equipment and software.

Recent applications of telemedicine cover activities such as remote consultations in specialties from dermatology to psychiatry, the transmission of electrocardiograms and radiological images, the provision of accident and emergency to offshore oil rigs, remote foetal monitoring, and education for health professionals (Currell *et al.*, 1997). The rapid developments in the technology are enabling healthcare organizations to construct new ways of providing healthcare. The current interest in telemedicine is supported by the proliferation of portable, affordable, desktop systems and the development of international telecommunications (Scannell *et al.*, 1995). The literature suggests a rapid expansion of telemedicine in North America (Scannell *et al.*, 1995) and in Europe (Wootton, 1995). However, this rapid pace of change suggests that proper evaluation of new applications may not be taking place, as there is evidence in the literature to indicate the need for rigorous assessment. As with any form of technology there is a need to assess the effectiveness, efficiency, equity and safety of telemedicine (see Chapter 5).

Breastfeeding and social support

Although pregnancy, childbirth and breastfeeding should be viewed as normal physiological processes, they can cause many major life changes and difficulties that may result in stress. Niven (1992) describes pregnancy, childbirth and the puerperum as a uniquely stressful life experience. Stress and anxiety can be reduced by the presence of good social support systems and networks. Social support plays an important role in the process where individuals adapt to major life changes and refers to the perceived comfort, caring, esteem or help a person receives from other people or groups (Lazarus and Folkman, 1984; Cohen, 1985). Social support may be defined as:

- emotional support (emotion-focused) which affirms that a person is accepted and valued and can relieve the emotional impact of the stressful situation by using thoughts and indirect actions
- informational support (problem-focused) which provides advice in understanding and coping with a stressful event by altering or managing the situation in an active and constructive way
- instrumental support (resource-focused) which provides assistance with money, resources or services.

Individuals use a range of specific responses to all three types, sometimes simultaneously and to varying degrees. There is no clear consensus regarding which type of support or coping strategy is most effective in maintaining positive mental health, because coping strategies have different consequences when used in response to different types of stress. In a study comparing the social support variables between women who had decided either to breastfeed or to bottle feed, it was found that women who intended to breastfeed had higher levels of informational support and were more active in seeking information than their bottle-feeding counterparts (Bell and Watson, 1997). However, there was no difference in the instrumental and emotional support available to either group.

Nurses, midwives and health visitors play a significant role in empowering mothers to grow into parenthood (Hodnett and Osborn, 1989; Hillan, 1992), and all forms of encouraging early contact between the mother and her newborn seem to have a favourable effect on the success of breastfeeding (Klaus and Kennel, 1970; Tamminen, 1989). However, professionals themselves must feel empowered with sufficient training and knowledge if they in turn are to empower women to breastfeed. Empowerment is defined as a process whereby individuals and communities gain mastery over their own lives (Rappaport, 1984). The negotiation of partnerships between midwives and breastfeeding mothers may be described as the first step in empowerment. Support after discharge from hospital is important, since, as stated previously, many women abandon this form of feeding when they face difficulties alone at home. Home-based support for these women has the potential to improve significantly the uptake of and duration time of breastfeeding. In systematic reviews, home-based support programmes have no known risks and may have important benefits for mothers and their babies (Hodnett and Roberts, 1997).

Randomized control trials (RCTs) and quasi-experimental designs

A clinical trial is defined as a prospective study comparing the efficacy of a test experiment or intervention against a control treatment in human subjects. Randomization is a procedure in which the play of chance enters into the assignment of a subject to a test situation or a control, so that assignment cannot be predicted in advance. Randomization also guarantees that statistical tests will have valid statistical levels. In the 1960s and 1970s many classic experiments of social psychology took place in the laboratory under controlled conditions and were open to criticism that they were totally unnatural (see Chapters 5 and 8, Stage 5).

Today, most RCTs take place in 'real life' settings. One major difficulty with this study design is that if subjects know that they are taking part in an experiment, they may knowingly or unknowingly wish to comply totally with the rules of the experiment. In other words, they will want to answer all questions the way that they think that the investigator expects them to, and this is known as the 'Hawthorne effect'. Because of this effect many experimenters attempt to conceal the purpose of the study from the subjects, and many argue that this is unethical and manipulating. In the following experiment the women in the sample knew exactly what was happening and it is worth noting that no harm was done to mother or baby and no one was subjected to stress or distress.

RCTs are often impossible in principle and quasi-experimental designs are used instead. This is a logically weaker paradigm, but it includes a comparison of groups, one receiving a 'treatment' and another acting as a 'control'. The design of the study is a pre- and post-test intervention which seeks to select equivalent groups through matching certain variables. Here the researcher tries to find subjects for a control group who will match the subjects of the experimental group.

Present study

The present study illustrated a quasi-experimental design with pre- and post-intervention groups: one group receiving the telemedicine link and a second acting as a control group receiving normal support mechanisms. The study was conducted from November 1998 to April 1999 in the maternity unit of a maternity hospital and in the subjects' own homes in the community (Lazenbatt et al., 2001a).

Aims and objectives

The aim of the study was to establish a telemedicine link in the homes of women who had decided to breastfeed, to provide informational, instrumental and emotional support. The study assessed whether use of the telemedicine technology as a support system facilitated and increased the duration of breastfeeding. The objectives of the study were to:

- test the effectiveness of the technology in supporting breastfeeding in comparison with a control group
- assess how the woman and her partner appraised the technology – whether they saw it as positive or negative, helpful or unhelpful
- assess if using the technology as a support system increased the duration of breastfeeding.

The following individuals comprising the research, hospital and community teams are shown in the box.

Research team	**Hospital and community team**
Acting chief executive, Community Trust	Hospital midwife manager and delivery suite
Programme manager – Mental Health,	manager
Community Trust	Senior nurse
Acting director of nursing, Community Trust	Community midwife manager
Director of the Institute of Telemedicine and	Hospital midwife/ lactation consultant
Telecare, University Hospital	Hospital midwife – postnatal
Lecturer, University	Hospital midwife – Neonatal Unit
R&D Research Fellow, University	Midwife – Neonatal Unit (night duty)
	Primary services coordinator
	Ward manager – Maternity Outpatients
	Breastfeeding advisor
	GP in the community
	Voluntary organizations – La Leche League

Subjects and methods

Timescale

The study was to assess and test the use of the technology over a 2–3-month period. The study used both qualitative and quantitative measures (see Chapters 5 and Chapter 8, Stages 5 and 6). The pre- and post-testing with quantitative attitudinal and knowledge questionnaires and topic guided semi-structured interviews were undertaken in the antenatal period (36–38 weeks) and 6–8 weeks postnatally (see Appendices 1 and 2).

Recruitment of the sample

Women who had decided in the antenatal period to breastfeed were initially approached about the study by the lactation consultant in the Maternity Unit. If the women agreed to take part in the study they were then contacted by the research team. The woman's experience of breastfeeding and the use of the technology had to be dealt with carefully. The confidentiality of the women and their partners was also guaranteed and ethical approval for the study was obtained. Women were recruited to the study if they were primiparous mothers and had decided to breastfeed during the antenatal period. All women were reassured that they would receive the usual breastfeeding support available at the hospital and in the community. Initially 10–12 women were required for the experimental group, but due to problems in obtaining the telemedicine equipment, only two machines were allocated to the study. The study wanted to select equivalent groups through matching by trying to find subjects for the experimental group who matched the subjects in the control group on certain variables. This allowed the study to exclude certain confounding variables by using specific selection criteria, which are listed below, for both the woman and her baby.

To be eligible for inclusion in the study a woman had to be:

- a primipara
- breastfeeding for the first time
- living with a partner
- aged 18–35 years
- a non-smoker
- not included in a high-risk group due to conditions such as diabetes, asthma, multiple birth, pre-term etc.
- delivering > 38 weeks
- delivering an infant of 2500 g and without any major problem.

To be eligible for inclusion in the study the baby had to be:

- put to the breast immediately after birth
- kept with the mother (rooming in) and not put in the nursery at night
- not offered complementary feeds or water
- delivered in a ward with no advertising or promotion of infant formula.

The study format was explained to all eligible women and their partners and consent was obtained antenatally (36–38 weeks). Four women meeting the above criteria were allocated to one of two groups:

1 *'Experimental' group*: these two women received the 'normal' support in hospital and the community that was given to the control group, and also received the telesupport link in their homes for 2–3 months.

2 *'Control' group*: these two women received 'normal' support with breastfeeding while in hospital and follow-up for 2–3 months (this included a telephone support service already in operation within the hospital).

Study design:
Timescale, interviews and measures

Stage 1: Antenatal Maternity Unit phase, 36–38 weeks
At the time of recruitment and before allocation the researchers conducted a semi-structured focus group interview with the women and their partners (both groups, four couples) in the Maternity Unit of the hospital to ascertain their knowledge and feelings towards breastfeeding and covered the following:

- general questions about pregnancy, birth, delivery and the decision to breastfeed, the duration of breastfeeding if they were working, any preconceived anxieties and worries
- feelings the women and their partners had about breastfeeding and its advantages and disadvantages
- whether the women and their partners recognized the need for support when breastfeeding.

All women and their partners were told that they would receive 'normal' hospital and community support for breastfeeding, which included the use of a telephone support service. Both groups of women and their partners completed pre-test Attitude to Breastfeeding and Knowledge of Breastfeeding questionnaires which were constructed for the study (see Appendices 1 and 2). Two women were then allocated to the experimental group and two to the control group. Both groups received their respective Breastfeeding Diary and were asked to complete it both antenatally for the rest of their pregnancy and for eight weeks postnatally (see Appendix 3).

Stage 2: Antenatal home phase, 38–41 weeks
Experimental group: The women and their partners had the technology installed in their homes and the telemedicine link demonstrated as a support system.

Stage 3: Postnatal home phase, 2–3 months
The experimental group and their partners were interviewed at home using a semi-structured interview schedule to assess the telemedicine link as a support system. They were also asked to assess breastfeeding success and to identify any problem areas or difficulties and to complete the post-test Attitude to Breastfeeding questionnaire. The 'control' group were also interviewed at home and asked to assess the nature of their success and support mechanisms and to identify any problem areas or difficulties.

Data collection and analysis

Data collection and analysis from the focus group were conducted in accordance with grounded theory (Strauss, 1990), allowing the concepts to be confirmed or modified as the study progressed. The framework method of data analysis and coding was applied throughout and themes were identified (Ritchie and Spencer, 1994). The language used by the women and their partners when they discussed breastfeeding was examined in detail using the principles of discourse analysis (Potter and Wetherell, 1995). The Attitude to Breastfeeding questionnaire had three response categories on a Likert type scale that ranged from 'yes' to 'not at all'. Each response was scored with higher scores reflecting a more positive attitude. The Knowledge of Breastfeeding questionnaire had five Likert style response categories that ranged from 'strongly agree' to 'strongly disagree'. Items for both of these questionnaires were based on evidence-based material and systematic reviews.

The breastfeeding diary

The use of diaries as a data collection method in health and social research has been increasing (Corti, 1993; Gibson, 1995). To monitor and record the nature of breast-feeding in the experimental group and in the control group, the study constructed self-completion baby feeding diaries (colour-coded for the two groups, pink (experimental) and white (control)). The diary was used as a research instrument, as it was seen as less invasive and more tactful for the collection of sensitive and intimate information. It allowed a woman to provide an account of her personal thoughts and feelings as well as being a useful log for events (see Appendix 3).

Every effort was made to make the diary as attractive as possible with regard to format and layout. In order to fulfil the function of a log and to make quantitative comparisons it had a semi-structured format. However, it was equally important that respondents were not guided to the point that they recorded only the type of information they thought the researchers wished to hear. Respondents were therefore instructed to record whatever was important to them. The diary questions were formulated on the basis of evidence of 'best practice' within breastfeeding research. The diary was divided into weekly sections followed by a blank page for further comments if the women or their partners wished to add anything (see Appendix 3).

Research midwives

The research midwives in the hospital were trained in using the telemedicine equipment (see Appendix 4). A room was set aside in the Maternity Unit for the exclusive use of the equipment and this allowed the midwife to communicate with the woman through the telelink with complete privacy and confidentiality. A protocol was developed (see Appendix 5) to allow the nursing staff to code the following information from the woman and her partner:

- the main reasons for using the telemedicine link
- the timing of the consultation (night or day)
- the nature of the woman's or her partner's needs (psychological or informational support)
- the woman's problems or questions (requests for symptom or pain control, positioning of the baby, cracked nipples, etc)
- the infant's problems (relief of crying, feeding regimes, colic, refusing to feed etc.)
- the duration of the consultation

- the support given, either informational or emotional, to the woman
- the support given, either informational or emotional, to the partner
- the picture and sound quality of the telelink
- limitations of the telemedicine link.

Results

Four women were recruited to the study and matched for certain variables, two were allocated to the telelink group and two to the control group. No statistically significant differences were seen in the other variables in the two groups. The duration of exclusive breastfeeding to date for those who received the telelink was eight weeks, compared with seven weeks in the control. At eight weeks both couples in the 'treatment' group asked to have the telemedicine machine removed from their houses because at this stage they were confident that they would continue to breastfeed until they resumed full-time employment. In one case the woman was a freelance artist whose timetable during the day permitted her to breastfeed until such time as she and the baby wished to stop. Both women in the control group felt competent with their ability to breastfeed and were also keen to continue until they returned to work.

Statistical analysis

Variables were compared between the control and intervention groups using the *t*-test for continuous variables and chi-square for categorical variables. Although the numbers in each group were small, statistical analyses were performed mainly as an illustration. In any experimental design larger numbers would be required to ascertain statistically significant differences, to provide validity and to exclude Type 1 error. Statistical analyses could include ANOVA to compare post-intervention scores from the two questionnaires. Logistic regression analysis could also be used to evaluate the impact of selected explanatory factors on the support mechanisms for breastfeeding.

After analyses there were no pre-treatment differences between the two groups on the Attitude and Knowledge questionnaires that were constructed specifically to measure a woman and her partner's knowledge about breastfeeding and the woman's attitude to breastfeeding (see Table 13.1).

Table 13.1 *t*-test differences in the Attitude to Breastfeeding questionnaire and the Knowledge of Breastfeeding questionnaire

	Intervention group (n=2)	Control group (n=2)
Attitude	48	50.5
Knowledge	88.5	81

Results from the Knowledge of Breastfeeding questionnaire (see Appendix 6)

Women in the intervention group   Both women either 'strongly agreed' or 'agreed' with all the beneficial statements: breastfeeding helps a woman regain her figure, it is best for baby and is inexpensive. However, one woman was unaware of the benefits with respect to breast cancer, ovarian cancer and osteoporosis. Both women were in agreement that it could be a painful process, sometimes difficult and that it could interfere with their sexual relationship. They disagreed that it is not for working women and that it would interfere with their social lives or their partner's relationship with the baby. With respect to the baby they unanimously 'strongly agreed' with all the benefits to baby.

Partner in the intervention group   Both partners 'agreed' and 'strongly agreed' with all the beneficial statements and appeared to be aware of all the major benefits of breastfeeding. They 'agreed' with the opinion that it could be painful and difficult and one partner felt it could be embarrassing and stressful while the other partner 'disagreed' with these statements. They 'disagreed' that it would affect their social lives or their relationship with the baby.

Women in the control group   Both women again 'strongly agreed' or 'agreed' with the beneficial statements: breastfeeding helps a woman get closer to her baby, it makes her feel more motherly and helps her to regain her figure. Worryingly, neither woman knew of the beneficial effects with respect to breast and ovarian cancer. They also 'disagreed' that it is not for working women, that it would affect their social lives or partner's relationship with the baby.

Partner in the control group   Both partners 'agreed' or 'strongly agreed' with the benefits of breastfeeding: it helps a woman get closer to her baby; it makes her feel more motherly; it is natural and best for the baby. However, both partners were unaware of the benefits with respect to breast and ovarian cancer and one partner 'disagreed' that it would be beneficial with osteoporosis or with a woman regaining her figure. They also 'agreed' with the opinion that it could be painful, embarrassing and stressful. They 'didn't know' about it being difficult or whether it could affect their sexual relationship.

Results from the Attitude to Breastfeeding questionnaire

There were no differences between the two groups both pre- and post-intervention on the Attitude questionnaire. The results showed that in both the experimental and control groups most support was being delivered to the mothers by their community midwives, health visitors or partners and extended family.

Diaries

The notes from the diaries, were carefully written by the research team. The wealth of information emerging from the diaries was too great to be included in this example but specific data referring to the telelink have been included below.

MOTHER 1 (JANE)

Jane made eight calls to the telelink and these ranged from 5 minutes to 35 minutes duration. Breastfeeding was witnessed as part of the normal lifestyle of Jane with her family and friends and she was therefore more confident in her own ability to breastfeed her baby. She felt unselfconscious in breastfeeding in front of other people and enjoyed its simplicity: as she said herself, 'No equipment necessary and the supply is always there!' Although confident, she didn't always enjoy feeding her baby and had some anxieties and fears about engorgement and mastitis.

Informational support   This mostly came from midwives in hospital and the community, her health visitor, and from family and friends. The lactation consultant through the telelink was a constant source of information and support. In week 1 she was able to reassure Jane and dispel any fears and anxieties, she was able to see the baby feeding and was initially pleased with the detail that the machine could pick up. In week 3 the link was of particular assistance one evening when the baby appeared to be crying constantly. The midwife suspected colic and she was able to demonstrate, visually with a doll, the positions in which Jane should hold the baby to increase its comfort. In week 4 Jane had a sore right breast and suspected that it was caused by a blocked duct. The lactation consultant could not see enough detail on the video screen to diagnose the problem and had to rely on Jane's description. She was able to demonstrate visually on a model of a breast the massage technique for relieving the problem, but advised Jane to come to the hospital the next day if she was still worried.

Instrumental support   Jane's partner offered consistent support not only with breastfeeding but also assisted with housework and making meals. As she had been very anaemic and run down during and after pregnancy she stayed with her mother in week 5 for extra help and support. Her mother helped a lot with the baby (bathing, dressing and taking her for a walk) which allowed Jane to get extra sleep.

Emotional support   The baby appears to have made this couple closer. In week 5 Jane was extremely anxious about her sore breast becoming mastitis. Her husband gave her the support she required by looking after the baby and reassuring her. By week 6 Jane felt that she had established a good feeding pattern and was more energetic.

Difficulties with the telelink
- Using the apparatus was difficult when holding the baby – it was much better when Jane's husband was at home to deal with the technical side.
- The picture was extremely bad on occasions and the midwife at the other end had to keep very still. Any movement caused the image to become blurred.
- The telelink machinery was cumbersome and unsightly and couldn't be moved easily around the house.
- The lactation consultant usually resorted to using the phone rather than the telelink as the delay in sound was extremely frustrating when trying to discuss a problem or attempting to support the mother.
- By week 8 Jane felt that she did not need the telelink and asked to have it removed from the house.

MOTHER 2 (MARY)

Mary used the telelink on three occasions and these ranged from 5 minutes to 12 minutes duration. Mary felt confident with breastfeeding even in the hospital and was really unsure if she needed the equipment. Breastfeeding was a normal occurrence in her extended family and she felt that she would receive sufficient support and encouragement from friends and relations. Mary initially called the telelink to show her health visitor how it operated.

Informational support   Again this mostly came from midwives in hospital and the community, her health visitor, and from family and friends. Mary felt that she had an excellent community midwife and therefore didn't need to use the telelink even though she was home from hospital after four days. However, in week 2 her community midwife diagnosed that she had mastitis. Mary at this stage used the telelink and found that the lactation consultant was a constant source of information and support. Her mastitis was treated very successfully by her community midwife and health visitor. In week 3 Mary called the team as the baby would not breastfeed and through the telelink the midwife was able to reassure Mary and dispel any fears and anxieties. She was able to see the baby feeding and was pleased with the detail that the machine could pick up. In week 4 Mary called the team again and told the research midwife that her baby would not breastfeed. Mary felt he was snuffly and was not able to feed and breathe effectively. The research midwife was able to see that Mary had very full breasts and suggested that she express some milk, and that she should place a cushion for support to enable Mary to get the baby correctly latched. Thanks to the telelink the midwife was able to observe the baby feeding well for 5 minutes and reassured Mary until she settled the baby.

Instrumental   Mary's initial confidence stemmed from the reassurance of extended family support. Although such help was forthcoming in the form of housework and others caring for the baby there were several occasions when Mary needed additional professional help which the research midwife was able to provide.

Emotional support   The baby appears to have made this couple closer. In week 4 Mary was extremely anxious about the baby's cold and ability to feed. Her husband provided support by looking after the baby and reassuring her and also helping her link with the research midwife. By week 7 Mary felt that she had established a good feeding pattern and no longer needed the telelink.

Difficulties with the telelink

- Using the apparatus was again difficult when holding a baby – it was much better when Mary's husband was there to assist her.
- The picture reception was poor and any movement caused the image to become blurred.
- Mary found the telelink machinery unsightly and disliked it sitting in her living room. She would have preferred it had it been easily portable.
- By week 7 Mary was confident with her feeding pattern and wanted the telelink removed from her house; she suggested that it could be used by someone else.

Discussion

This quasi-experiment was undertaken to assess, in an unbiased fashion, whether or not introducing a home-based telelink increases the duration of breastfeeding for up to two months among mothers who start exclusive breastfeeding. The aim of the study was not to promote the initiation of breastfeeding. The results show that the telelink alone was not responsible for increasing the duration when given to primiparous mothers who breastfed from birth. Both of the mothers in the telelink group stated that they had used the machinery, but judged that it was unsightly and had limited portability. They also reported that they had difficulty in positioning themselves and their baby in front of the machinery. More importantly, communication through the machine was extremely difficult in that the sound quality was poor and the picture often became erratic if either party moved at all. These difficulties meant that meaningful communication by means of the link became torturous and both mothers disliked using the machine.

However, the greatest advantage of the machine was that it allowed both mothers to contact and gain support from the lactation consultant at the hospital. They felt that she gave most support and information even though she usually had to revert to using the phone to communicate with the mothers. Both mothers also had an excellent support system from their community midwives who they felt offered all the assistance that was required. However, one woman in the treatment group stated that she felt the machine helped in a 'crisis' point in breastfeeding. The telelink contact with the hospital was in the middle of the night and contact with the midwife reassured both mother and partner and allowed the baby to resume feeding.

Characteristics of the study site and sample, as well as features of the study design, should be considered in interpreting the results. The maternity unit, in which the study was conducted, is strongly committed to breastfeeding. Secondly, the study participants had to be reduced to two as the research team had difficulties in receiving a larger number of 'telemedicine' machines. This small number did not allow for any comparable analyses and weakened the validity of results. Thirdly, all women in the sample were primiparous and breastfed their babies at hospital discharge. With this selection criteria for the study none of the women received a commercial formulae package or had a low birthweight baby. Therefore two known risk factors for shortening breastfeeding were not present (Richardson and Champion, 1992; Dungy, 1994). All these features may explain why the women in both groups are still breastfeeding their babies.

There are two possible explanations for the results. The first is that the hospital has an excellent verbal counselling and advice approach to breastfeeding in their routine maternity service and this support and communication may have established a plateau of duration which cannot be increased easily with the use of the telelink. The second is that the telelink alone is not sufficient as it is well known that breastfeeding practice is influenced not only by knowledge, but also by many social and psychological factors as well as by close contact with well trained health professions. Both mothers in the telelink group highlighted the unnatural style of communication it produced, both with poor sound and limited picture. For them the significant support was obtained just as well by telephone contact with the lactation consultant, but the personal contact from the community midwife was the most beneficial and supporting (Lazenbatt et al., 2001a).

RCTs and quasi-experimental designs provide the most compelling evidence of efficacy. When searching the literature there appears to be no other experimental design which measures the efficacy of a telelink to promote the initiation or duration of breastfeeding. However, the results of this study suggest that the efficacy of a telelink alone in prolonging breastfeeding is very limited among those mothers who are already breastfeeding at discharge. In the future, the study could be replicated with a larger sample of higher risk mothers known to avoid breastfeeding, such as those who are from disadvantaged or from more isolated areas. Although this style of study and the machinery is costly, in both equipment and in professional contact, the research team feel that the telelink would prove more beneficial if it was used in conjunction with linkages to other breastfeeding mothers (peer support) and also further links with collaborating voluntary agencies such as La Leche League and the National Child-birth Trust.

Outcomes

Immediate outcomes

- The results from the Knowledge questionnaire suggest that women and their partners need more education with respect to the beneficial effects of breastfeeding on breast and ovarian cancer, as well as its effects on osteoporosis. The effect that breastfeeding may have on the couple's sexual relationship should also be highlighted.
- Although this study had serious limitations and restrictions, it is important that negative findings are reported in any evaluation and disseminated widely. Every evaluation should highlight what works and what does not appear to work so that recommendations can be made in the future.
- The results suggest that women are losing personal contact and support through the telelink – informational support can be given over the telelink but emotional and instrumental support were less obvious.

Intermediate outcomes

- The study suggests that there is a need to introduce policies into the workplace that would allow a longer duration for breastfeeding, including longer maternity leave for women, as all of the mothers were suggesting that they would terminate breastfeeding when they returned to work. The introduction of better working conditions is essential as this is perhaps the most significant variable to interfere with the duration of breastfeeding.

Longer-term outcomes

- Studies such as this may in the longer term assist the hospital in attaining Baby-Friendly Status, which would be the first such award in Northern Ireland. Indeed, inequalities in health could be reduced for mother and baby alike: for the infant increased natural immunities and health advantages; for the mother increased protection from breast and ovarian cancer as well as an impact on osteoporosis (Lazenbatt et al., 2001a).

Success Indicators	Outcome

1   APPROACHES/PARTNERSHIPS

Health alliances/inter-agency
Evidence suggests that lack of professional effectiveness has been shown to be one of the first barriers to successful breastfeeding. Gordon (1998) suggests that it is the historical medicalization of childbirth in Northern Ireland and control of infant nutrition that has resulted in rigid hospital routines and practices. Indeed, voluntary organizations such as the National Childbirth Trust and La Leche have brought to light the neglect of breastfeeding in some hospitals.

Multidisciplinary
The failure of medical, midwifery and nursing staff to provide sufficient equitable support and encouragement was identified as a major factor militating against successful breastfeeding for mothers.

2   TOOLS (METHODS)

Audit/evaluation
The rapid pace of change with technology suggests that proper evaluation of new applications such as telemedicine may not be taking place. There is evidence in the literature to indicate the need for rigorous assessment of these new technologies. As with any form of technology there is a need to assess the effectiveness, efficiency, equity and safety of telemedicine. Although this study had serious limitations and restrictions, it is important that negative findings are reported in any evaluation and disseminated widely. Every evaluation should highlight what works and what does not appear to work so that recommendations can be made in the future.

Research
A clinical trial is defined as a prospective study comparing the efficacy of a test experiment or intervention against a control treatment in human subjects. Randomization is a procedure in which the play of chance enters into the assignment of a subject to a test situation or a control, so that assignment cannot be predicted in advance. Randomization also guarantees that statistical tests will have valid statistical levels. In the 1960s and 1970s many classic experiments of social psychology took place in the laboratory under controlled conditions and were open to the charge that they were totally unnatural. The study assessed whether use of the telemedicine technology as a support system facilitated and increased the duration of breastfeeding. It illustrated a quasi-experimental design with pre-and post-intervention groups: one group receiving the telemedicine link, and a second acting as a control group receiving normal support mechanisms.

3   RESOURCES

Setting
The study was conducted from November 1998 to April 1999 in the Maternity Unit of the Ulster Hospital and in the subjects' own homes in the community. Support after discharge from hospital is important, since, as stated previously, many women abandon this form of feeding when they face difficulties alone at home. Home-based support for these women has the potential to improve significantly the uptake of and duration time of breastfeeding. In systematic reviews, home-based support programmes have no known risks and may have important benefits for mothers and their babies.

Support materials
The present study assessed the use of a telemedicine link within the maternity hospital as such a support system for mothers. The technology involved was intended to act as a support system or peer network to prolong the duration of breastfeeding in the community. The use of telemedicine has been reported in a variety of forms, from the 1960s onwards. The rapid developments in technology are enabling healthcare organizations to construct new ways of providing healthcare.

Delivery agent
The UNICEF baby-friendly initiative is a global campaign run jointly with the World Health Organization (WHO) to raise breastfeeding rates. The initiative encourages hospitals to strive towards and achieve ideal quality standards. Attaining Baby-Friendly Status is a significant challenge for many hospitals. Nurses, midwives and health visitors play a significant role in empowering mothers to grow into parenthood. However, professionals themselves must feel empowered with sufficient training and knowledge in order for them to empower women to breastfeed.

Training delivery agent
Hospitals have to implement a 10-step plan for successful breastfeeding covering everything from staff training to rooming-in, artificial teats and complementary feeding policies. In addition, they should have a success rate of 50% of mothers who are still breastfeeding at time of discharge. To date, only three hospitals have achieved Baby-Friendly Status; all stress that they provide appropriate support for mothers, but their major challenge is to extend the duration of the women's breastfeeding.

4   INDIVIDUAL/COMMUNITY

Holistic health
Many studies have explored the reasons why women stop breastfeeding and have concluded that there are a variety of factors which may affect this. These include physical factors such as sore and cracked nipples, perceived insufficient milk supply, lack of professional and social support, limited antenatal education/knowledge. Hospital policies/midwifery practices and psychological factors such as attitudes to breastfeeding may also influence a woman's decision to discontinue. However, there is evidence to

suggest that several of these problems might be prevented if health professionals were to show mothers how to position the baby correctly and to offer higher levels of practical and emotional support to the mother.

Culture
The prevalence of breastfeeding has declined in many parts of the world for a variety of social, economic and cultural reasons. Social class, age, smoking habit and the age at which the mother completed full-time education are all related to the incidence of breastfeeding. Its incidence is higher among women from higher social classes, older first-time mothers, non-smokers and those who have continued education beyond the age of 18 years. In addition, birth order influences breastfeeding, with rates highest among first-time mothers. The feeding method chosen for the first child also influences how subsequent siblings are fed.

Empowerment
Not all mothers may wish to convert to breastfeeding, but those who wish to do so should be empowered and facilitated by midwives and nurses. Empowerment is defined as a process whereby individuals and communities gain mastery over their own lives. The negotiation of partnerships between midwives and breastfeeding mothers may be described as the first step in empowerment. However, several studies suggest that health professionals have relatively little influence on a woman's decision relating to feeding. The WHO suggests that, unwittingly, health services may have contributed to the decline in breastfeeding by either failing to support and empower mothers to breastfeed or by introducing routines and procedures that interfere with its establishment.

APPENDIX 1

Attitudes to breastfeeding questionnaire

		Yes	Sometimes	Not at all
1.	Do you like the new shape of your body?	_____	_____	_____
2.	Do you think that your partner finds you sexually desirable?	_____	_____	_____
3.	Do you feel anxious about feeding your baby?	_____	_____	_____
4.	Do you worry that you may not be a good mother?	_____	_____	_____
5.	Does your partner support you when needed?	_____	_____	_____

6. Do you find the new shape of your breasts attractive?   _____   _____   _____

7. Do you think you will feel in control of breastfeeding?   _____   _____   _____

8. Do you feel happy and contented about breastfeeding?   _____   _____   _____

9. Do you feel unattractive?   _____   _____   _____

10. Do midwives and health visitors support you with breastfeeding?   _____   _____   _____

11. Do you think that your relationship with your partner will change if you breastfeed your baby?   _____   _____   _____

12. Do you wish to feed your baby immediately after birth?   _____   _____   _____

13. Do you want to breastfeed for a certain period of time?   _____   _____   _____

14. Do you have a good sexual relationship with your partner?   _____   _____   _____

15. Do you think that breastfeeding is better than bottle feeding?   _____   _____   _____

16. Do you think that breastfeeding could stop you from having a social life?   _____   _____   _____

17. Do you feel depressed at the moment?   _____   _____   _____

18. Do you think that you will breastfeed when you return to work?   _____   _____   _____

19. Do your family and friends support you when needed?   _____   _____   _____

20. Do books and magazines provide you with information?   _____   _____   _____

APPENDIX 2

Knowledge of Breastfeeding: Women's questionnaire

Breastfeeding is good for you as a woman because it:
(Please **tick** the answer which most applies to you)

	Don't know	Disagree	Strongly disagree	Strongly agree	Agree
Helps reduce the risk of breast cancer and ovarian cancer	_____	_____	_____	_____	_____
Helps reduce the risk of bone disease in later life	_____	_____	_____	_____	_____
Helps a woman feel more motherly	_____	_____	_____	_____	_____
Helps a woman regain her figure	_____	_____	_____	_____	_____
Helps a woman get closer to her baby	_____	_____	_____	_____	_____
Helps a woman feel sexy	_____	_____	_____	_____	_____
Is inexpensive	_____	_____	_____	_____	_____
Is natural	_____	_____	_____	_____	_____
Is the best for your baby	_____	_____	_____	_____	_____

Breastfeeding is not so good for you as a woman because it:
(Please **tick** the answer which most applies to you)

	Don't know	Disagree	Strongly disagree	Strongly agree	Agree
Is sometimes a painful process	_____	_____	_____	_____	_____
Is sometimes difficult	_____	_____	_____	_____	_____
Is embarrassing	_____	_____	_____	_____	_____

Is tiring and stressful ___ ___ ___ ___ ___

Is not for women who are
working ___ ___ ___ ___ ___

May interfere with your
social/family life ___ ___ ___ ___ ___

May interfere with your
partner's relationship with
the baby ___ ___ ___ ___ ___

May interfere with your
sexual relationship ___ ___ ___ ___ ___

May make your other
children jealous ___ ___ ___ ___ ___

May mean that you should
give up smoking ___ ___ ___ ___ ___

May mean that you should
give up drinking alcohol ___ ___ ___ ___ ___

Breastfeeding is good for your baby because it:
(Please **tick** the answer which most applies to you)

	Don't know	Disagree	Strongly disagree	Strongly agree	Agree
Is more beneficial to a baby's health	___	___	___	___	___
Is more beneficial to premature babies	___	___	___	___	___
Helps reduce the risk of chest and ear infections	___	___	___	___	___
Helps reduce the incidence of gastroenteritis in babies	___	___	___	___	___
Helps reduce the risk of allergies	___	___	___	___	___

Breastfeeding may not be so good for your baby because it:
(Please **tick** the answer which most applies to you)

	Don't know	Disagree	Strongly disagree	Strongly agree	Agree
May interfere with your partner's involvement with the baby					
May interfere with other family member's involvement with the baby					
Is really no better than bottle feeding your baby					
May make baby's weight gain appear slow					

Knowledge of Breastfeeding: Partner's questionnaire

Breastfeeding is good for a woman because it:
(Please **tick** the answer which most applies to you)

	Don't know	Disagree	Strongly disagree	Strongly agree	Agree
Helps reduce the risk of breast cancer and ovarian cancer					
Helps reduce the risk of bone disease in later life					
Helps a woman feel more motherly					
Helps a woman regain her figure					
Helps a woman get closer to her baby					

Helps a woman feel sexy	___	___	___	___	___
Is inexpensive	___	___	___	___	___
Is natural	___	___	___	___	___
Is the best for the baby	___	___	___	___	___

Breastfeeding is not so good for a woman because it:
(Please **tick** the answer which most applies to you)

	Don't know	Disagree	Strongly disagree	Strongly agree	Agree
Is sometimes a painful process	___	___	___	___	___
Is sometimes difficult	___	___	___	___	___
Is embarrassing	___	___	___	___	___
Is tiring and stressful	___	___	___	___	___
Is not for women who are working	___	___	___	___	___
May interfere with your social/family life	___	___	___	___	___
May interfere with her partner's relationship with the baby	___	___	___	___	___
May interfere with her sexual relationship	___	___	___	___	___
May make her other children jealous	___	___	___	___	___
May mean that you should give up smoking	___	___	___	___	___
May mean that you should give up drinking alcohol	___	___	___	___	___

Breastfeeding is good for your baby because it:
(Please **tick** the answer which most applies to you)

	Don't know	Disagree	Strongly disagree	Strongly agree	Agree
Is more beneficial to a baby's health	_____	_____	_____	_____	_____
Is more beneficial to premature babies	_____	_____	_____	_____	_____
Helps reduce the risk of chest and ear infections	_____	_____	_____	_____	_____
Helps reduce the incidence of gastroenteritis in babies	_____	_____	_____	_____	_____
Helps reduce the risk of allergies	_____	_____	_____	_____	_____

Breastfeeding may not be so good for your baby because it:
(Please **tick** the answer which most applies to you)

	Don't know	Disagree	Strongly disagree	Strongly agree	Agree
May interfere with your involvement with the baby	_____	_____	_____	_____	_____
May interfere with other family member's involvement with the baby	_____	_____	_____	_____	_____
Is really no better than bottle feeding your baby	_____	_____	_____	_____	_____
May make baby's weight gain appear slow	_____	_____	_____	_____	_____

APPENDIX 3

Breastfeeding diary

Name _____

Weeks 1–8

How is breastfeeding this week?

_____ These questions
_____ might help you
_____ when completing
_____ your diary
_____
_____
_____ Has breastfeeding
_____ been successful,
_____ easy or difficult,
_____ or had problems?
_____
_____
_____ Have you had many
_____ problems – mastitis,
_____ cracked nipples,
_____ baby crying?
_____
_____
_____
_____ Are you sleeping
_____ well?
_____ Is baby sleeping
_____ well?
_____
_____
_____ Are you feeling OK?
_____ Is baby well?
_____
_____
_____
_____ Does your partner
_____ like you to
_____ breastfeed?

_____
_____
_____
_____
_____   Does breastfeeding
_____   make you feel more
_____   like a woman?
_____
_____
_____
_____
_____   Does it interfere
_____   with life?
_____
_____

Weeks 1–8

Are you getting support with breastfeeding?

_____   These questions
_____   might help you
_____   when completing
_____   your diary
_____
_____
_____
_____   Your partner gives
_____   a lot of support
_____
_____
_____
_____   Your family and
_____   friends are very
_____   supportive
_____
_____
_____   No one supports
_____   you, especially at
_____   night
_____
_____

_____   Midwives, health
_____   visitors are helpful
_____
_____
_____
_____
_____   No one can really
_____   support you
_____
_____
_____
_____
_____   Outside agencies are
_____   helpful
_____
_____
_____
_____
_____

Weeks 1–8

*Experimental group only

**What did you use the telesupport machine
for this week?**

_____   These questions
_____   might help you
_____   when completing
_____   your diary
_____
_____
_____
_____   What sorts of things
_____   did you use the
_____   machine for – baby/
_____   mother problems?
_____
_____
_____
_____   Did you use it every
_____   day or just now and
_____   again?

_____
_____
_____
_____
_____   What time of day
_____   did you use it most
_____   and for how long?
_____
_____
_____
_____   Do you think it
_____   provided you with
_____   support?
_____
_____
_____
_____   Did your partner
_____   find it helpful?
_____
_____
_____
_____   Limitations of link
_____   picture, sound etc.
_____
_____
_____
_____

APPENDIX 4

Telemidwifery calls

1   Link mothers will contact the breastfeeding advisor or on-call midwife by dialling
    —— —— and asking switchboard to bleep ——.
2   The person who answers the bleep will return the call by using the telemidwifery
    equipment in the breastfeeding advisor's office.
3   Connect the equipment as follows:
    First remove the small white telephone socket and replace with the dark
    grey lead for the telelink phone and placing it back into the same socket
    marked 2171. Make sure the machinery is plugged in (white socket and
    lead).

4   Make your call and afterwards document any details using the Research Protocol Record Sheet.

5   Before leaving the office replace the telephone socket for the Breastfeeding Helpline answerphone.

6   Please remember to hand in your bleep and the office key to SCBU before going off duty.

*In case of difficulties contact lactation consultant at home on —— —— or mobile ——.

APPENDIX 5

Research protocol for telelink calls

Name of caller: _____

Date and time of call (day or night) _____

Main reason for using telelink _____

Nature of the woman's or partner's needs e.g. practical, psychological, informational support _____

Woman's problems, e.g. perceived or true milk insufficiency, painful breasts or nipples, pain control, positioning, questioning, cracked nipples, engorgement, blocked ducts, mastitis, thrush, stress, distress, lack of sleep etc. _____

_____

Infant problems, e.g. excessive crying, frequent feeding, refusing to feed, colic, inadequate weight gain etc. _____

_____

Partner's problems, e.g. distress, stress, information, needs support etc.

_____

Duration of the consultation _____

Support given and to whom, e.g. informational or emotional to woman and partner

_____

Any limitations of telelink e.g. picture and sound quality, interaction with client etc.

_____

APPENDIX 6

Women's and partners' responses to Knowledge of Breastfeeding questionnaire

Women's responses: intervention group (n=2)

Breastfeeding is good for you as a woman because it:	SA (%)	A (%)	DK (%)	D (%)	SD (%)
Helps a woman regain her figure	50	50			
Helps a woman get closer to her baby	100				
Helps reduce the risk of breast cancer and ovarian cancer		50	50		
Helps reduce the risk of bone disease in later life		50	50		
Helps a woman feel more motherly	100				
Helps a woman feel sexy		50	50		
Is inexpensive	50	50			
Is natural	100				
Is the best for your baby	100				

Breastfeeding is not so good for you as a woman because it:	SA (%)	A (%)	DK (%)	D (%)	SD (%)
Is sometimes a painful process		100			
Is sometimes difficult		100			
Is embarrassing				50	50
Is tiring and stressful		50		50	
Is not for women who are working				100	
May interfere with social/family life				50	50
May interfere with your partner's relationship with the baby				50	50
May interfere with your sexual relationship		100			
May mean that you should give up smoking		100			
May mean that you should give up drinking alcohol		50		50	

Breastfeeding is good for your baby because it:	SA (%)	A (%)	DK (%)	D (%)	SD (%)
Is more beneficial to a baby's health	100				
Is more beneficial to premature babies	100				
Helps reduce the risk of chest and ear infections	100				
Helps reduce the risk of gastroenteritis in babies	100				
Helps reduce the risk of allergies	100				

Breastfeeding is not so good for your baby because it:	SA (%)	A (%)	DK (%)	D (%)	SD (%)
May interfere with your partner's involvement with baby		50			50
May interfere with other family member's involvement with baby		50			50
Is really no better than bottle feeding your baby					100
May make baby's weight gain appear slow				50	50

Partner's responses: intervention group (n=2)

Breastfeeding is good for a woman because it:	SA (%)	A (%)	DK (%)	D (%)	SD (%)
Helps a woman regain her figure	50	50			
Helps a woman get closer to her baby	100				
Helps reduce the risk of breast cancer and ovarian cancer		100			
Helps reduce the risk of bone disease in later life		100			
Helps a woman feel more motherly	50	50			
Helps a woman feel sexy		100			
Is inexpensive		100			
Is natural	100				
Is the best for your baby	100				

Breastfeeding is not so good for a woman because it:	SA (%)	A (%)	DK (%)	D (%)	SD (%)
Is sometimes a painful process		100			
Is sometimes difficult		100			
Is embarrassing		50		50	
Is tiring and stressful		50		50	
Is not for women who are working			100		
May interfere with social/family life				100	
May interfere with your partner's relationship with the baby				100	
May interfere with your sexual relationship			100		
May mean that you should give up smoking		100			
May mean that you should give up drinking alcohol		100			

Breastfeeding is good for your baby because it:	SA (%)	A (%)	DK (%)	D (%)	SD (%)
Is more beneficial to a baby's health	100				
Is more beneficial to premature babies		50	50		
Helps reduce the risk of chest and ear infections			100		
Helps reduce the risk of gastroenteritis in babies		50	50		
Helps reduce the risk of allergies			100		

Breastfeeding is not so good for your baby because it:	SA (%)	A (%)	DK (%)	D (%)	SD (%)
May interfere with your partner's involvement with baby		50			50
May interfere with other family member's involvement with baby				100	
Is really no better than bottle feeding your baby				50	50
May make baby's weight gain appear slow			50	50	

Women's responses: control group (n=2)

Breastfeeding is good for you as a woman because it:	SA (%)	A (%)	DK (%)	D (%)	SD (%)
Helps a woman regain her figure		100			
Helps a woman get closer to her baby	100				
Helps reduce the risk of breast cancer and ovarian cancer			100		
Helps reduce the risk of bone disease in later life			100		
Helps a woman feel more motherly	100				
Helps a woman feel sexy			50	50	

	SA (%)	A (%)	DK (%)	D (%)	SD (%)
Is inexpensive		100			
Is natural	100				
Is the best for your baby	100				

Breastfeeding is not so good for you as a woman because it:	SA (%)	A (%)	DK (%)	D (%)	SD (%)
Is sometimes a painful process		100			
Is sometimes difficult		50	50		
Is embarrassing				100	
Is tiring and stressful		100			
Is not for women who are working				100	
May interfere with social/family life				50	50
May interfere with your partner's relationship with the baby				50	50
May interfere with your sexual relationship	50	50			
May mean that you should give up smoking		100			
May mean that you should give up drinking alcohol		50		50	

Breastfeeding is good for your baby because it:	SA (%)	A (%)	DK (%)	D (%)	SD (%)
Is more beneficial to a baby's health	100				
Is more beneficial to premature babies	50		50		
Helps reduce the risk of chest and ear infections		100			
Helps reduce the risk of gastroenteritis in babies		100			
Helps reduce the risk of allergies	50	50			

Breastfeeding is not so good for your baby because it:	SA (%)	A (%)	DK (%)	D (%)	SD (%)
May interfere with your partner's involvement with baby		50	50		
May interfere with other family member's involvement with baby		50			50
Is really no better than bottle feeding your baby					100
May make baby's weight gain appear slow				50	50

Partner's responses: control group (n=2)

Breastfeeding is good for a woman because it:	SA (%)	A (%)	DK (%)	D (%)	SD (%)
Helps a woman regain her figure		50	50		
Helps a woman get closer to her baby	100				
Helps reduce the risk of breast cancer and ovarian cancer			100		
Helps reduce the risk of bone disease in later life			50	50	
Helps a woman feel more motherly	50	50			
Helps a woman feel sexy			50	50	
Is inexpensive			100		
Is natural	100				
Is the best for your baby	100				

Breastfeeding is not so good for a woman because it:	SA (%)	A (%)	DK (%)	D (%)	SD (%)
Is sometimes a painful process		100			
Is sometimes difficult			100		
Is embarrassing		100			

	100				
Is tiring and stressful	100				
Is not for women who are working			50	50	
May interfere with social/family life			50	50	
May interfere with your partner's relationship with the baby				100	
May interfere with your sexual relationship			100		
May mean that you should give up smoking	50	50			
May mean that you should give up drinking alcohol	50	50			

Breastfeeding is good for your baby because it:	SA (%)	A (%)	DK (%)	D (%)	SD (%)
Is more beneficial to a baby's health	100				
Is more beneficial to premature babies		100			
Helps reduce the risk of chest and ear infections			100		
Helps reduce the risk of gastroenteritis in babies			100		
Helps reduce the risk of allergies			100		

Breastfeeding is not so good for your baby because it:	SA (%)	A (%)	DK (%)	D (%)	SD (%)
May interfere with your partner's involvement with baby				50	50
May interfere with other family member's involvement with baby				100	
Is really no better than bottle feeding your baby				100	
May make baby's weight gain appear slow			100		

FURTHER READING

Basire, K. (1997) Baby-feeding: the thoughts behind the statistics. *New Zealand Medical Journal*, 110 (1044): 184–7; May 23, 121–128.

Bell, C. and Watson, L. (1997) An initiative to promote and support breastfeeding. *Health Visitor*, August, 70(8): 294–296.

Buckner, E. (1993) Support networks utilization by breastfeeding mothers. *Journal of Human Lactation*, 9: 231–235.

Cohen, S. (1985) Stress, social support and the buffering hypothesis. *Psychological Bulletin*, 98 (2): 310–317.

Cole, J. (1977) Breastfeeding in the Boston suburbs in relation to personal-social factors. *Clinical Paediatrics*, 16: 352–356.

Corti, L. (1993) Using diaries in social research. *Social Research Update*, 2:1–6.

Currell, R., Urquhart, C., Wainwright, P. and Lewis, R. (1997) *A Systematic Review of the Impact of Telemedicine as an Alternative to Face-to-Face Patient Care, on Professional Practice and Patient Care.* York: The Cochrane Library, Issue 4.

DHSS (1994) *Maternal and Child Health: An Action Plan.* HPSS, Northern Ireland.

DHSS (1997) *Health and Wellbeing into the Next Millennium: a Regional Strategy for Health and Social Wellbeing 1997–2002.* Northern Ireland.

Dungy, C.I. (1994) Maternal attitudes as predictors for infant feeding decisions. *Journal of the Association Acad Minor Phys*, 5:159–164.

Foster, K., Lader, D. and Cheesborough, S. (1997) *Infant Feeding Survey 1995.* London: HMSO.

Freed, L. (1994) Effect of expectant mothers' feeding plans on the prediction of fathers' attitudes regarding breastfeeding. *American Journal of Perinatology*, 10: 300–303.

Gibson, A. (1995) An analysis of the use of diaries as a data collection method. *Nurse Researcher*, 3(1): 66–73.

Gordon, M. (1998) Empowerment and breastfeeding, in S. Kendall (ed.) *Health and Empowerment*. London: Arnold.

Graffy, J.P. (1992) Mothers' attitudes to and experience of breastfeeding: a primary care study. *British Journal of General Practice*, 42: 61–64.

Hillan, E.M. (1992) Issues in the delivery of midwifery case. *Journal of Advanced Nursing*, 17(3): 274–278.

Hillervik, C. and Hofvander Sjoln, S. (1977) Factors relating to early termination of breastfeeding. *Acta Paediatrica Scandinavia*, 66: 505–511.

Hodnett, E.D. and Osborn, I. (2000) *Home-based Social Support for Socially Disadvantaged Mothers*. Cochrane Database of Systematic Reviews, Issue 2, p. CD000107.

Hodnett, E.D. and Roberts, I. (1997) *A Systematic Review of Home-based Social Support for Socially Disadvantaged Mothers*. The Cochrane Library, Issue 4.

Horton, S. (1996) Breastfeeding promotion and priority setting in health. *Health Policy and Planning*, 11(2): 156–168.

Inch, S. (1996) Breast milk and formula milk: what's the difference. *Midars Midwifery Digest*, March, 6(1): 80–84.

Inch, S. and Renfrew, M.J. (1989) Common breastfeeding problems. In I. Chalmers (ed.) *Effective Care in Pregnancy and Childbirth*. Oxford: Oxford University Press.

Jones, D.A. (1984) Breast feeding problems. *Nursing Times*, 80(33): 53–54.

Jones, D.A. (1986) Attitudes of breastfeeding mothers: a survey. *Social Science and Medicine*, 23:1151–1156.

Jones, D.A. and West, R.R. (1986) Effect of a lactation nurse on the success of breastfeeding: a randomized control trial. *Journal of Epidemiology and Community Health*, 40: 45–49.

Kendall, S. (1995) Cross-cultural aspects and breastfeeding promotion. *Health Visitor*, 68: 450–451.

Klaus, M.H. and Kennell, J.H. (1970) Parent Infant Bonding. St Louis: Mosby.

Kvist, L.J., Persson, E. and Lingman, G.K. (1996) A comparative study of breastfeeding after traditional postnatal hospital care and early discharge. *Midwifery*, 12: 85–92.

Lazarus, R.S. and Folkman, S.M. (1984) *Stress and Coping*. London: Harcourt Brace.

Lazenbatt, A. (2000) Tackling inequalities in health in Northern Ireland. *Community Practitioner*, 73(2): 481–483.

Lazenbatt, A. and Hunter, P. (2000) 'An evaluation of a drop-in centre for working women'. Queen's University of Belfast/Royal College of Nursing, Northern Ireland.

Lazenbatt, A. and Orr, J. (2001) Evaluation and effectiveness in practice. *International Journal of Nursing Practice*, 7(6) (in press).

Lazenbatt, A., McWhirter, L., Bradley, M. and Orr, J. (1999) The role of nursing partnership interventions in improving the health of disadvantaged women. *Journal of Advanced Nursing*, 30(6): 1280–1288.

Lazenbatt, A., McWhirter, L., Bradley, M. and Orr, J. (2000a) Community nursing achievements in targeting health and social need. *Nursing Times Research*, 5(3): 178–192.

Lazenbatt, A., McWhirter, L., Bradley, M., Orr, J. and Chambers, M. (2000b) Tackling inequalities in health and social wellbeing – evidence of 'good practice' by nurses, midwives and health visitors. *International Journal of Nursing Practice*, 6(2) April: 76–88.

Lazenbatt, A., Sinclair, M., Salmon, S. and Calvert, J. (2001a) Telemedicine as a support system to encourage breastfeeding in Northern Ireland: a case study design. *Journal of Telemedicine and Telecare* (in press).

Lazenbatt, A., Lynch, U. and O'Neill, E. (2001b) Revealing the hidden 'troubles' in Northern Ireland: the role of Participatory Rapid Appraisal. *Health Education Research* (in press).

Libbus, M.K. (1992) Perspectives on common breastfeeding problems. *Journal of Human Lactation*, 8(4): 199–203.

Libbus, MK. (1994) Perceptions of breastfeeding and infant feeding choice in a group of low income Mid-Missouri Women. *Journal of Human Lactation*, 10:17–23.

Lynch, M., Blair, J. and Jones, V. (1986) Infant feeding decisions among women from a population in Georgia. *Journal of the American Dietetic Association*, 90: 250–259.

Moore, R., Mason, C., Harrisson, S. and Orr, J. (1997) *An Assessment of Health Inequalities in Two Northern Ireland Communities: An Ethnographic Approach*. DHSS (NI).

Morgan, E. (1985) *The Descent of Women*. London: Souvenir Press.

Niven, C.A. (1992) *Psychological Care for Families Before, During and After Birth*. London: Heinemann.

Oakley, A. and Rajan, L. (1993) What did your baby eat yesterday? Social factors and infant feeding practices. *European Journal of Public Health*, 3(1): 18–27.

Office of National Statistics (1997) *Infant Feeding 1995*. London: HMSO.

Potter, J. and Wetherell, M. (1995) Analysing discourse. In A. Bryman and R.G. Burgess (eds) *Analysing Qualitative Data*, pp. 47–66. London: Routledge.

Purtell, M. (1994) Teenage girls' attitudes to breastfeeding. *Health Visitor*, 67(5):156–157.

Rajan, L. (1993) The contribution of professional support, information and consistent correct advice to successful breastfeeding. *Midwifery*, June 2, 197–209.

Rappoport, J. (1984) Studies in empowerment: introduction to the issue. *Prevention in Human Services*, 3: 1–7.

Rea, M.F., Venancio, S.I. and Batista, L.E. (1997) The possibilities and limitations of breastfeeding among women in formal employment. *Revista de Saude Publica*, 31(2): 149–156.

Richardson, V. and Champion, V. (1992) The relationship of attitudes, knowledge and social support to breastfeeding. *Issues in Comprehensive Paediatric Nursing*, 15: 183–197.

Ritchie, J. and Spencer, L. (1994) Qualitative data analysis for applied policy research. In A. Bryman and R.G. Burgess (eds) *Analysing Qualitative Data*, pp. 173–194. London: Routledge.

Scannell, K., Douglas, A., Perednia, M. and Kissman, H. (1995) Telemedicine: past, present and future. *Current Bibliographies in Medicine*. Maryland: National Library of Medicine.

Selye, H. (1978) *Stress in Health and Disease*. London: Butterworth.

Strauss, A. (1990) *Basics of Qualitative Research: Grounded Theory Procedures and Techniques*. London: Sage.

Voss, S., Finnis, L. and Manners, J. (1993) Fathers and breastfeeding: a pilot observational study. *Journal of the Royal Society of Health*, 113:176–178.

White, A., Freeth, S. and O'Brien, M. (1992) *Infant Feeding 1990 Office of Population Censuses and Surveys*. London: HMSO.

WHO/UNICEF (1989) *Protecting, Promoting and Supporting Breastfeeding: the special role of maternity services*. Geneva: WHO.

Wiles, L.S. (1984) The effect of prenatal breastfeeding education on breastfeeding success. *Journal of Obstetric, Gynaecological and Neonatal Nursing*, 13: 253–257.

Wootton, R. (1995) *TeleMed 95 Telemedicine on the Superhighway*. London: Royal Society of Medicine Press.

Wylie, J. and Verber, I. (1994) Why women fail to breastfeed? *Journal of Nutrition and Dietetics*, 7:115–120.

GLOSSARY

Assessment   Estimation of the relative magnitude, importance or value of needs observed.

Clinical governance   Involves health professionals wanting to assure the quality and accountability of their healthcare delivery. This requires staff not only to work in partnerships, breaking down boundaries by providing integrated care within health and social care teams, but also to participate fully in audit and evaluation programmes.

Community   In modern societies, especially highly urban societies, individuals rarely belong to a single distinct community but maintain membership of a range of communities based on variables such as geography, occupation, social contact, values and other important features of their lives; e.g. gay community, hearing and non-hearing communities.

Community development   Refers to the process of facilitating communities' awareness of the factors and forces which affect their health and quality of life, and ultimately helping to empower them with the skills needed for taking control over and improving those conditions in their community which affect their health and way of life. It often involves helping them to identify issues of concern and facilitating their efforts to bring about change in these areas.

Community empowerment   Community empowerment includes a raised level of psychological empowerment among the community members, with a political action component in which they have actively participated, and the achievement of some redistribution of resources favourable to the community or group in question.

Community organization   Linking community groups and structures and residents together over common issues and helping to facilitate organizational efforts to bring about change.

Community participation (community involvement)   Involving people in the processes which affect their health. Some people use this term to refer to involving people in health promotion activities. Others use it to refer to involvement in decision-making structures that affect health, including intersectoral approaches to community health planning and promotion. Most effective participation occurs when a community's skills have been developed (community development), that is, when a community is skilled in the processes of participation and decision-making.

Comparison group   A group of people with similar characteristics to the participants in a health programme, but who do not receive the programme. The two groups are compared over time, as a measure of programme effects.

Control group   A type of comparison group, where the people are allocated to the experimental group or the comparison group at random. That is, the two groups are drawn randomly from the same population.

Decision-makers   People who make decisions about the allocation of resources for existing and future programmes; those people to whom reports evaluating health programmes are usually submitted, e.g. health administrators, representatives of government or funding bodies.

Effectiveness   The ability of an intervention to achieve its intended effect in those to whom it is offered, that is, its ability in practice or effect in the real world. Effectiveness concerns the question 'Does it work?'

Efficacy   The ability of an intervention to achieve its intended effect in those individuals who comply under optimal conditions; effect in an ideal world. Efficacy concerns the question 'Can it work?'

Efficiency   The effectiveness of a programme (improvement in health) in relation to costs (in terms of time, labour, material consumed). Participant discomfort or other costs may be taken into account. Note: sometimes used to refer only to costs, without considering outcome.

Empowerment   Empowerment comes to fruition within a person and enables that person to recognize his or her own dignity and autonomy and to reflect this in drawing up his or her own health promotion agenda.

Epidemiology   The study of the distribution and determinants of health-related states and events in human populations. Traditionally this study has been applied to the control of disease, but it is now increasingly applied to disease prevention and health promotion.

Equity   Equity in health means (WHO, 1986) that ideally everyone should have a fair opportunity to attain their full health potential and, more pragmatically, that no one should be disadvantaged from achieving this potential if it can be avoided.

Evaluation   The process by which we decide the worth or value of something. For health promotion, this process involves measurement and observation (evaluation research) and comparison with some criterion or standard (usually a programme goal).

Evaluation research   Observations and measurements made for the purpose of evaluation.

Experimental group   A group of people involved in an experiment who receive an intervention, as compared with the comparison group, who receive no intervention. Allocation into groups is ideally by random assignment.

Formative evaluation   Evaluation for the purpose of improving the programme as it is being implemented.

Goal (health goal)   The desired long-term outcome of a health intervention, such as a reduction in the health problem or improvement in health status.

Health   An important resource for living; physical abilities and social and psychological capacities to achieve one's potential and respond positively to the challenges of the environment.

Health attitude   A view or way of thinking about health or health behaviour. For example, if knowledge refers to the awareness that the rate of breast cancer is high among women who smoke, attitude might refer to the desire to decrease one's chances of contracting cancer as well as the intention to stop smoking.

Health behaviour (health-directed behaviour) Any activity undertaken by an individual with the intention of maintaining, protecting or promoting health, whether or not the activity is effective for that purpose.

Health-related behaviour Any activity undertaken by an individual which has been shown to have a positive or negative effect on health, whether or not such activity is carried out with any intention towards health.

Health belief A statement or thought, declared or implied intellectually and/or emotionally accepted as true by a person or group. May motivate behaviour related to health.

Health education Consciously constructed opportunities for learning which are designed to facilitate voluntary changes in behaviour towards a predetermined goal. It is closely associated with disease prevention and involves changing behaviours which have been identified as risk factors for particular diseases. Targets individuals and groups, organizations and communities.

Health impact assessment Identifies those activities and policies likely to have major impacts on the health of a population. It is thought of as a group of research activities such as evaluation, partnership working, public consultation, and quality assurance and utilization indicators as well as available evidence for more explicit decision-making.

Health intervention Any planned action which is aimed at reducing a health problem by intervening in the existing causal chain. An intervention is the sum of all the strategies; that is, those events, circumstances or materials which directly involve the target group or the community.

Health knowledge The information that an individual has, or has access to, which provides the basis for attitude and decisions about health, health behaviour and risk behaviour.

Health promotion The process of enabling individuals and communities to increase control over the determinants of health and thereby improve their health. Health promotion grew out of the health education movement, but can now be understood as an umbrella concept which covers health education and a number of other approaches aimed at changing living conditions and lifestyles for the purpose of promoting health.

Health services Refers to the organized provision of healthcare by health professionals both in the public and private sectors. Examples: hospitals, community health centres, specialist medical and paramedical services such as physiotherapy, occupational therapy.

Health status State of physical and/or mental and /or social functioning. The literature on health status measurement for the most part predates the concern with quality of life, but some measures incorporate aspects now thought of as affecting quality of life.

Impact evaluation Follows evaluability assessment in the steps of programme evaluation and is the first step in testing a completed programme's performance. Impact evaluation is concerned with the immediate effects of the programme, that is its effect on those factors which contribute to or cause the health problem in question. Corresponds to the measurement of programme objectives. Should include an assessment of both intended and unintended effects.

Intersectoral   In health promotion health-orientated policy affecting and involving sectors outside the health service (such as employment, housing, food production, social care), but usually evolved in collaboration with the health sector. Also used to refer to collaboration between different levels of various sectors, e.g. government health authorities plus local transport authority plus community education.

Intervention group   Any collection of individuals participating in a health programme or intervention. In most cases the intervention group consists of those who will directly benefit (target group) or a subset of this group. In some cases a programme may be directed at one group of people for the benefit of another group, e.g. in drug education for parents the parents are the intervention group but the children are the target group.

Morbidity   Illness episodes. Morbidity data describe the prevalence of different diseases and other health problems in the community. The main source of this is hospital admission records which include diagnosis or reason for admission. Data collected by GPs, health centres and others may also be included.

Mortality   Death. Mortality data on causes and number of deaths per year are collected by the Registrar General.

Need   Health needs are understood as being those states, conditions or factors that, if unmet, prevent people from achieving optimum physical, mental, social and environmental health. This would include such things as minimum provision of basic health services and information, a safe physical environment, good food and housing, productive work and activity and a network of emotionally supportive and stimulating relationships.

Needs assessment   The initial step in planning any health intervention; the process of identifying and analysing the priority health problem and the nature of the target group, for the purpose of planning an intervention.

Network   A set of relationships which centres on one individual's circle of contacts and branches outward to include relationships between these people and others already in the network.

Networking   In health promotion this refers to the building up of the quantity and quality of one's relationships and making use of one's social or professional network for the purpose of generating or receiving information or support.

Objective   A defined result of specific activity to be achieved in a finite period of time by a specified person or number of people. Objectives state who will experience what change or benefit by how much and by when.

Outcome evaluation   The final phase of programme evaluation and the second of the two-step process which tests the performance of a programme. Outcome evaluation answers the question of whether a programme has achieved its goal; whether it has been able to reduce the health need or alleviate the problem isolated at the needs assessment stage, and at what cost. It also corresponds to the measurement of programme goals, whereas impact evaluation corresponds to the measurement of programme objectives. In this regard outcome evaluation is concerned with longer-term effects than those addressed in impact evaluation.

Perceived health   An individual's interpretation of experiences of health and ill health within the context of everyday living. This judgment is normally based on available knowledge and information modified by previous experience and social and cultural norms.

Process evaluation   Process evaluation is the first element of programme evaluation. It measures the activity of the programme and who it is reaching. It determines to what extent a programme has been implemented as planned, by measuring (a) programme reach, (b) participant satisfaction, (c) implementation of programme activities, (d) performance of materials or other components, and (e) on-going quality assurance. Process evaluation includes pre-testing of materials or other components of the programme and may lead to the redesign or re-implementation of programme elements. See *formative evaluation*.

Programme   A coherent series of activities which together make up strategies to be carried out with a group of participants for the purpose of improving the health status of the target group. This can be individual behaviour change, or environmental, legislative or other change. A programme is usually planned in response to an established health need. The word is used synonymously with intervention.

Programme evaluation   Assessment of programme effectiveness; determination of the value or degree of success of a programme in achieving set goals and objectives and the assessment of unintended effects.

Psychological empowerment   Psychological empowerment is a feeling of greater control over one's own lives which individuals experience through group membership and may occur without participation in collective political action.

Qualitative data   Data which describe the range of response and variation between responses but do not record the frequency of response. Cannot be used with tests of statistical significance.

Quantitative data   Data which are recorded as frequency of response; response options may be categorical (e.g. male/female); ordinal (e.g. never/sometimes/often); or numerical (number of cigarettes smoked per day). Hypotheses may be supported or rejected by applying tests of statistical significance to quantitative data.

Randomized control trial (RCT) (equivalent group designs)   Random assignment gives all participants an equal chance of being allocated to the experimental group or the control group. The groups are compared by pre-testing and post-testing or by time series testing. This design is classified as the true experiment and is considered the strongest design for demonstrating causality.

Reliability   A property of questionnaires, surveys and other measurement tools. Expresses the degree to which the same score is produced on repeated measures with a given measurement, in the absence of any real change. Repeated measures refers to measurements taken with the same instrument either by the same person at different times (test–retest reliability) or by different people (inter-observer reliability).

Risk factor   Any aspect of behaviour, society or environment which is directly linked to a health problem in an established or proposed causal pathway. A health problem may have one or more than one risk factor, e.g. smoking and elevated levels of serum cholesterol are both risk factors for heart disease.

Social support   Social support is known to have a direct and positive effect upon health and wellbeing and is also known to be a buffer against stressful life events. There are different types of assistance which an individual is able to obtain from people with whom they come into contact, e.g. emotional support; instrumental support (which includes the provision of money, goods and services, and assistance with everyday tasks); informational support; and appraisal (meaning feedback to the individual about their identity, personality and behaviour).

Strategy   A plan of action that anticipates barriers and resources in relation to achieving a specific objective.

Summative evaluation   Questions about whether the programme has met its objectives or its intended effects.

Survey   An investigation in which information is systematically collected from a population sample, e.g. face-to-face inquiry, self-completed questionnaire or telephone survey.

Target group   Those members of a community for whose benefit a health goal is constructed and a health intervention carried out. These people are usually the programme participants or intervention group.

Users of evaluation   Those people or bodies that will make use of programme evaluations for the purpose of health planning and resource allocation.

Validity   A property of questionnaires, surveys, or any other research measurement tool. Expresses the degree to which the tool measures what it purports to measure e.g. to what extent a questionnaire can be a valid measure of smoking status.

FURTHER READING

General poverty

Fyfe, G. (1994) *Poor and Paying for it: The Price of Living on a Low Income*. London: HMSO/Scottish Consumer Council.

Hills, J. (1993) *The Future of Welfare: A Guide to the Debate*. York: Joseph Rowntree Foundation.

Mack, J. and Lansley, S. (1985) *Poor Britain*. London: Allan and Unwin Press.

Mack, J. and Lansley, S. (1991) *Breadline Britain in the 1990s*. London: Harper Collins.

National Childrens Bureau (1990) *Child Poverty and Deprivation in the UK*. London: National Childrens Bureau.

Oppenheim, C. (1993) *Poverty: The Facts*, revised and updated edition. London: Child Poverty Action Group.

Oppenheim, C. and Harker, L. (1996) *Poverty: The Facts*, revised and updated edition. London: Child Poverty Action Group.

Robbins, D. (1994) *Observatory on National Policies to Combat Social Exclusion*. Copenhagen: Commission of the European Communities Directorate General V.

Roll, J. (1992) *Understanding Poverty: A Guide to Concepts and Measures*. London: Family Policy Studies Centre.

Sinfield, A. (1993) *Poverty, Inequality and Justice*. Social Policy Series No 6, Department of Social Policy and Social Work: University of Edinburgh.

Strathclyde Poverty Alliance (1994) *Communities against Poverty – a Resource Pack*. Glasgow: Strathclyde Regional Council.

Thake, S. and Staubach, R. (1993) *Investing in People – Rescuing Communities from the Margin*. York: Joseph Rowntree Foundation.

Poverty and health

Benzeval, M., Judge, K. and Whitehead, M. (1995) *Tackling Inequalities in Health: An Agenda for Action*. London: Kings Fund.

Blackburn, C. (1991) *Working with Families*. Buckingham: Open University Press.

Cole-Hamiliton, I. (1991) *Poverty can seriously Damage your Health*. London: Child Poverty Action Group.

Conway, J. (1988) *Prescription for Poor Health – the Crisis for Homeless Families*. London: London Food Commission, The Maternity Alliance, SHAC, Shelter.

Smith, R. (1987) *Unemployment and Health – A Disaster and a Challenge*. Oxford: Oxford University Press.

Lazenbatt, A., McWhirter, L., Bradley, M. and Orr, J. (1999) The role of nursing partnership interventions in improving the health of disadvantaged women. *Journal of Advanced Nursing*, 30(6): 1280–1288.

Lazenbatt, A., McWhirter, L., Bradley, M. and Orr, J. (2000) Community nursing achievements in targeting health and social need. *Nursing Times Research*, 5(3): 178–192.

Lazenbatt, A., McWhirter, L., Bradley, M., Orr, J. and Chambers, M. (2000) Tackling inequalities in health and social wellbeing – evidence of 'good practice' by nurses, midwives and health visitors. *International Journal of Nursing Practice*, 6(2) April: 76–88.

Lazenbatt, A. (2000) Tackling inequalities in health in Northern Ireland. *Community Practitioner*. 73(2): 481–483.

Lazenbatt, A. and Hunter, P. (2000) 'An evaluation of a drop-in centre for working women'. QUB/Royal College of Nursing, Northern Ireland.

Lazenbatt, A., Sinclair, M., Salmon, S. and Calvert, J. (2001) Telemedicine as a support system to encourage breastfeeding in Northern Ireland: a case study design. *Journal of Telemedicine and Telecare* (in press).

Lazenbatt, A. and Orr, J. (2001) Evaluation and Effectiveness in Practice. *International Journal of Nursing Practice*, 7(6) (in press).

Lazenbatt, A., Lynch, U. and O'Neill, E. (2001) Revealing the hidden 'troubles' in Northern Ireland: the role of Participatory Rapid Appraisal. *Health Education Research* (in press).

Townsend, P., Whitehead, M. and Davidson, N. (1992) *Inequalities in Health*. London: Penguin.

Wilkinson, R.G. (ed.) (1986) *Class and Health* London: Tavistock.

Wilkinson, R.G. (1994) *Unfair Shares: The Effects of Widening Income Differences on the Welfare of the Young*. London: Barnardo's.

Health promotion

Blaxter, M. (1990) *Health and Lifestyles*. London: Routledge.

Jacobson, B., Smith, A. and Whitehead, M. (1991) *The Nations Health*. London: King Edward's Hospital Fund.

Rodmell, S. and Watt, A. (1986) *The Politics of Health Promotion*. London: Routledge and Kegan Paul.

Cancer

Wilkinson, G.S. and Wilson, J. (1983) An evaluation of demographic differences in the utilization of cancer information service. *Social Science and Medicine* 17: 169–175.

Food

Leather, S. (1992) *Less Money – Less Choice: Poverty and Diet in the UK*. London: National Consumer Council HMSO.

National Children's Home (1991) *NCH Poverty and Nutrition Survey*. London: National Children's Home.

National Food Alliance (1994) *Food and Low Income: A Practical Guide for Advisors and Supporters of People on Low Incomes*. London: National Food Alliance.

Travellers

Fay, R. (1995) *Report on the Travellers' Health Project*. Dublin: Dublin Travellers' Education and Development Group.
Hennink, M. (1995) *Primary Health Care Needs of Travelling People in Wessex*. Working Paper, Department of Social Statistics, University of Southhampton.

Ethnic minorities

National Health Service in Scotland (1994) *Access to Health Care by the Ethnic Communities: a Guide to Good Practice*. Scotland: HMSO.
Sheldon, T. and Parker, H. (1992) Race and ethnicity in health research. *Journal of Public Health Medicine*, 14(2): 104–110.
Smage, C. (1995) *Health and Ethnicity: A Critical Review*. London: Kings Fund/SHARE.

Housing

Bhatti, M., Brooke, J. and Gibson, M. (1994) *Housing and the Environment: A New Agenda*. London: Chartered Institute of Housing.
Crofton, J. (1994) *Housing and Health Report*. Scotland: Shelter.
Hopton, J. (1996) The health effects of improvements to housing – a longitudinal study. *Housing Studies*, 11(2): 271–286.

Homelessness

Connelly, J. (1994) *Homelessness and Ill Health*. London: Royal College of Physicians.
Gaulton-Berks, L. (1994) Homeless choices. *Nursing Times*, 90(34): 52–54.

Collaboration

Fieldgrass, J. (1992) *Partnerships in Health Promotion: Collaboration between the Statutory and Voluntary Sectors*. HEA/ Wessex: Institute of Public Health Medicine.
Speller, N. and Funnell, R. (1994) *Towards Evaluating Healthy Alliances*. HEA/Wessex: Institute of Public Health Medicine.

Substance abuse

Bottomly, T. (1995) Peer education amongst crack users, not so cracked. *Druglink*, May/June, 9–12.
Power, R. (1994) *Some Methodological and Practical Implications of Employing Drug Users as Fieldworkers*. London: Taylor and Francis.

Evaluation

Baker, M. and Kirk, S. (1996) *Research and Development for the NHS: Evidence, Evaluation and Effectiveness*. Oxford: Ratcliffe Medical Press.

Bury, T. and Mead, J. (1998) *Evidence-based Healthcare: A Practical Guide for Therapists*. London: Butterworth-Heinemann.

Chalmers, I. and Altman, D.G. (1995) *Systematic Reviews*. London: BMJ Publishing Group.

Crump, B.J. and Drummond, M.F. (1993) *Evaluating Clinical Evidence: A Handbook for Managers*. Harlow: Longman.

Dixon, R. and Munro, J. (1997) *Evidence-based Medicine: A Practical Workbook for Clinical Problem-solving*. London: Butterworth-Heinemann.

Entwistle, V., Watt, I.S. and Herring, J. (1996) *Information about Healthcare Effectiveness: An Introduction for Consumer Health Information Providers*. London: King's Fund.

Greenhalgh, T. (1997) *How to Read a Paper*. London: BMJ Publishing Group.

Jadad, A. (1997) *Randomised Control Trials: A User's Guide*. London: BMJ Publishing Group.

Hawe, P. (1990) *Evaluating Health Promotion: A Health Worker's Guide*. Sydney: McLennan and Petty.

Jones, R. and Kinmouth, A.L. (1995) *Critical Reading for Primary Care*. Oxford: Oxford University Press.

Peckham, M. and Smith, R. (1996) *Scientific Basis of Health Services*. London: BMJ Publishing Group.

Sackett, D.L. (1991) *Clinical Epidemiology: A Basic Science for Clinical Medicine*. 2nd ed. Boston: Little Brown and Company.

Sackett, D.L. (1996) *Evidence-based medicine: How to Practice and Teach EBM*. London: Churchill Livingstone.

Community

Barr, A. (1996) Assessing community needs. *Scottish Journal of Adult and Continuing Education*, 1(1).

Barr, A., Hamilton, R. and Purcell, R. (1996) *Learning for Change*. London: Community Development Foundation.

Barr, A. (1996) *Practicing Community Development – Experience in Strathclyde*. London: Community Development Foundation.

Bell, J. (1992) *Community Development Teamwork: Measuring the Impact*. London: Community Development Foundation.

Bell, J. (1992) *A Framework for Evaluation in the Community and Voluntary Sectors*. London: Community Development Foundation.

Bryant, R. and Bryan, B. (1982) *Change and Conflict: A Study of Community Work in Glasgow*. Aberdeen: Aberdeen University Press.

Bryden, J., Watson, D., Storey, C. and van Alphen, J. (1995) *Community Involvement and Rural Policy*. Aberdeen: The Arkleton Trust.

Burns, R. and Black, M. (1989) A practical example of community participation. *Belfast Health Promotion*, 4(2).

Chanan, G. (1992) *Out of the Shadows: Local Community Action and the European Community*. Dublin: European Foundation for the Improvement of Living and Working Conditions, Shankill.

Chanan, G., Smithies, J. and Webster, G. (1995) *Local Project Monitoring and Evaluation Scheme*. London: Community Development Foundation / Labyrinth Training and Consultancy.

Chanan, G. and Mos, K. (1990) *Social Change and Local Action: Coping with Disadvantage in Urban Areas*. Dublin: European Foundation for the Improvement of Living and Working Conditions, Shankill.

Community Development Review Group (1991) *A Report on Education and Training for Community Development in Northern Ireland*. Belfast: Workers Educational Association.

Community Development Review Group (1991) *Perspectives for the Future*. Belfast: Workers Educational Association.

Community Development Review Group (1992) *Community Development in Northern Ireland: A perspective for the Nineties*. Belfast: Workers Educational Association.

Women

Action on Smoking and Health (1993) *Her Share of Misfortune – Women, Smoking and Low Income*. London: Action on Smoking and Health.

Elstad, J.I. (1996) Inequalities in health, related to women's marital, parental and employment status – a comparative study. *Social Science and Medicine*, 42(1): 75–89.

Glendenning, J. and Millar, J. (1987) *Women and Poverty in Britain*. London: Wheatsheaf.

Graham, H. (1993) *Hardship and Health in women's lives*. London: Harvester Press.

Webb, E. (1995) Sexual mores: female genital mutilation – a worldwide problem. *British Journal of Sexual Medicine*, 22(6): 6–8.

SOURCES OF FURTHER INFORMATION

Organizations concerned with clinical effectiveness

Charities Aid Foundation
Kings Hill, West Mailing,
Kent ME19 4TA.
Telephone: 01732 520000

Cochrane Collaboration
PO Box 726, Oxford OX2 7UX.
Telephone: 01865 310138
Fax: 01865 516311
E-mail: secretariat@cochrane.co.uk
(Systematic reviews of health-care
research)

Community Practitioners and Health
Visitors Association
50 Southwark Street, London SE1 1UN.
Telephone: 0207 717 4000
Fax: 0207 717 4040
(Advice, resource materials and practice
guidelines)

Critical Skills Appraisal Programme
PO Box 777, Oxford OX3 7LF.
Telephone: 01865 226986
Fax: 01865 226959
E-mail: casp@cix.compulink.co.uk

English National Board for Nursing,
Midwifery and Health Visiting
Victory House, 170 Tottenham Court
Road, London W1P 0HA.
Telephone: 0207 388 3131

Fax: 0207 383 4031
(Advice, resource materials and practice
guidelines)

Health Publications Unit
Two-Tem Communications
Wetherby LS23 7LN.
Telephone: 0541 555455 (NHS response
line)
Fax: 01937 845381

King's Fund Development Centre
(PACE programme)
11–13 Cavendish Square, London
W1M 0AN.
Telephone: 0207 307 2694
Fax: 0207 307 5810
E-mail: hhutton@kehf.org.uk
Web: www.kingsfund.org.uk
(Promoting Action on Clinical
Effectiveness (PACE))

National Co-ordinating Centre for
Health Technology Assessment
Boldrewood, University of Southampton,
Highfield, Southampton SO16 7PX.
Telephone: 01703 595586
Fax: 01703 595639
E-mail: hta@soton.ac.uk
Web: www.soton.co.uk/wi/hta
(Commissions and monitors research on
health technologies)

NHS Centre for Review and
Dissemination
University of York, Heslington, York
YO1 5DD.
Telephone: 01904 433648
Fax: 01904 433644
Email: crdpub@york.ac.uk
Web: http://www.york.ac.uk/list/crd/
info.htm
(Systematic reviews of specific health-
care interventions)

NHS Library Adviser
Skipton House, London.
Telephone: 0207 972 5921

Royal College of Midwives
15 Mansfield Street, London W1M 0BE.
Telephone: 0207 8725100
Fax: 0207 3123536
(Advice, resource materials and practice
guidelines)

Royal College of Nursing
20 Cavendish Square, London W1M
0AB.
Telephone: 0207 409 3333
Fax: 0207 730 7263
E-mail: fons@aial.pipex.co
(Advice and material on research in
nursing)

Journals that publish articles on clinical audit, clinical effectiveness and quality in healthcare

Audit Trends
Editor: Richard Baker
Eli Lilly National Clinical Audit Centre,
Department of General Practice and
Primary Health Care, University of
Leicester, Leicester
General Hospital, Gwendolen Road,
Leicester LE5 4PW.
Telephone: 0116 258 4873
Fax: 0166 258 4982
E-mail: clinaudit@le.ac.uk

British Medical Journal
BMA House, Tavistock Square,
London WC1 9JR.
Telephone: 0207 387 4499
Fax: 0207 383 6668
E-mail: 10032.1411@compuserve.com

Journal of Clinical Effectiveness
Editors: Gifford Batstone and Mary
Edwards
JCE, FT Healthcare Maple House,

149 Tottenham Court Road, London
W1P 9LL.
Telephone: 0207 274 3476
(answerphone only)

Network (the newsletter of the Clinical
Audit Association)
Editor: Patricia Kent
The Clinical Audit Association, Room 8,
Cleethorpes Centre, Jackson Place,
Wilton Road, Humberston, South
Humberside DN36 4AS.
Telephone/Fax: 01472 210682

Quality in Health Care
Editor: Fiona Moss
BMJ Publishing Group,
BMA House, Tavistock Square,
London WC1H 9JR.
Telephone: 0207 383 6204
Fax: 0207 383 6668
E-mail: 101317.475@compuserve.com

INDEX